Clinical Success

in

Immediate Complete Dentures:

An Alternative Approach

Michel Pompignoli, DCD, DSO

Private Practice
Paris, France

Former Assistant Professor
Department of Dental Surgery
University of Paris 5
Paris, France

Michel Postaire, DCD, DSO

Professor
Department of Dental Surgery
University of Paris 5
Paris, France

Didier Raux

Former Director, Dental Laboratory
Department of Dental Surgery
University of Paris 5
Paris, France

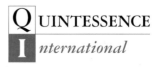

Paris, Berlin, Chicago, Tokyo, London, Milan, Barcelona,
Istanbul, São Paulo, Mumbai, Moscow, Prague, and Warsaw

First published in French in 2004 by Quintessence International, Paris: *La prothèse complète immediate*.
English translation by Jay K. Weiss, DMD.

ISBN 978-2-912550-57-6

Quintessence International
11 bis, rue d'Aguesseau
75008 Paris
France

Design: STDI, Lassay-les-Châteaux, France
Printing and Binding: EMD, Lassay-les-Châteaux, France

Printed in France

Acknowledgments

The authors wish to thank:

Professor J.-C. Thibault for the quality of his surgical procedures.

Dr P. Leroy for his contributions to the patient's prosthetic treatment.

Table of Contents

Preface

Becoming Completely Edentulous

When multiple extractions are indicated, a patient must undergo the transition of having all, or at least some, of his or her teeth to a new reality of being completely edentulous. Many treatment techniques have been developed to address patients' functional as well as psychologic and social needs and to facilitate this difficult transition by minimizing difficulties. These methods may be classified into two groups.

The Provisional Prosthesis

The emergency prosthesis

Because an emergency prosthesis is most frequently constructed in response to an unexpected emergency, it usually does not provide any of the elements that help patients transition into a new situation with fewer natural teeth. An emergency prosthesis is made to fit an existing clinical situation and usually involves simply adding prosthetic teeth to a pre-existing removable partial denture.

The emergency prosthesis should rarely be fabricated, because modifying an existing partial denture can:

- *Contribute to any pathologic state associated with the use of the prosthesis.*
- *Provide poor esthetics.* The added teeth and artificial gingiva rarely match the existing prosthesis. Such defects are frustrating and provide little comfort to patients facing edentulism. Patients cannot be psychologically prepared for a complete denture if they begin to fret about losing their last tooth.
- *Inhibit proper function.* Added teeth can never fully integrate into the original metallic base of a removable partial denture. Their presence, therefore, prevents the prosthetic equilibrium required for the proper performance of oral functions.
- *Cause resorption of the alveolar ridge.* Retaining periodontally mobile teeth for too long results in the iatrogenic loss of osseous structure and leaves a blunted alveolar ridge that cannot fully support or effectively stabilize a future complete denture.
- *Change the maxillomandibular relationship.* Too often modified partial dentures fail to preserve the vertical occlusion, which irreversibly dislocates the articulation and complicates the eventual construction of a complete denture.

The transitional prosthesis

If there is no emergency, the existing partial denture can serve as a provisional therapeutic device to prepare patients for edentulism. This functional re-adaptive prosthesis is particularly valuable when practitioners are not yet fully acquainted with their patient's functional parameters.

It is, therefore, indicated to:

• Re-establish stable, functional maxillomandibular relationships
• Prepare a denture base that will provide maximum support for complete dentures
• Retrain the neuromuscular and articulation functions
• Determine the correct denture size for the patient
• Prepare the patient psychologically for edentulism

In order to give patients the reassuring option of returning to their original clinical situation, a practitioner can create a duplicate of the existing prosthesis upon which all modifications and adjustments can be made.

The construction of a transitional prosthesis requires a lengthier time line to allow the clinical situation to adjust to the therapeutic prosthesis. This increases the treatment cost, and the provisional prosthesis will have to be replaced with a definitive prosthesis.

The complete provisional prosthesis

This denture is usually made quickly using approximate impressions taken shortly before or after the patient's last teeth have been extracted. The practitioner must estimate both the maxillomandibular relationship and the esthetics.

In order not to injure the supporting tissues, this provisional prosthesis is made of a "supple" material that requires frequent replacement. The practitioner can ensure an adequate occlusion only by a severe grinding-in of its artificial teeth.

This type of restoration causes tissue resorption and encourages patients to acquire habits that inhibit adaptation to the definitive complete denture. In addition to considerable increases in treatment cost, this technique forces the practitioner to devote time to adjustments and modifications as opposed to following a coherent clinical technique. Just as with an emergency prosthesis, it meets none of the quality criteria needed to help a patient transition toward complete edentulism. There are sufficient difficulties associated with the provisional prosthesis for both the patient and the practitioner to call its therapeutic utility into question.

The Immediate Complete Denture

Definition

This prosthodontic concept consists of placing a complete denture immediately after the extraction of the last teeth of a dental arch. This treatment takes into account the biologic and physiologic factors necessary for prosthetic integration. It helps patients to maintain or restore oral functions during the transition period. The aim of this prosthetic tool is to replace the patient's lost teeth as effectively as possible.

Objective

The treatment plan preserves the patient's remaining teeth, particularly the maxillary anterior dentition, during all phases of prosthetic preparation, including impression taking, registration of jaw relationships, construction of wax-ups, and fabrication of the dentures, until the prosthesis can be delivered.

Fabrication steps
- Construct a working cast based on all available clinical data needed for fabrication of the denture (ie, anatomic, functional, and esthetic).
- Modify the cast in accordance with esthetic goals as well as anticipated changes in bone and mucosa following surgical healing.
- Construct a surgical guide that will ensure that tooth extractions and any surgery at edentulous sites will harmonize with prosthetic needs.

Although patients are threatened by the loss of any of their remaining teeth, the psychologic trauma is greater when anterior teeth are involved. Complete maxillary edentulism occurs more frequently than complete mandibular edentulism, and the loss of the maxillary anterior incisors causes, by far, the greatest emotional trauma. When a patient suffers this kind of psychologic distress, dentists are not usually equipped to deal with it. Practitioners may be well advised to seek assistance from a psychotherapist. In such clinical situations, dentists should carefully assess their technical expertise and limitations to make sure they will be able to respond to the expectations of their patients without compromise.

> Complete edentulism is a handicap. Patients perceive it as an amputation, and dentists must provide them with the best possible therapeutic assistance to help them transition.

Clinical indications
This prosthesis is indicated for patients who are partially edentulous in the maxilla and require extraction of the six anterior teeth (or even extending to include the first premolars). The posterior maxilla must already be stable enough for supporting a prosthesis.

It is somewhat more difficult to construct an immediate denture for the mandible: Dentists find that stabilization of the denture base, which is required for proper healing, is harder to attain. Making a successful immediate denture simultaneously for both the maxilla and mandible is even more difficult.

Perspectives
The development and innovation of implant dentistry has considerably transformed prosthetic strategies. In treating completely edentulous jaws, dentists must always consider implants for both removable as well as fixed prostheses. However, the use of implants in no way changes the difficulty of shepherding a patient toward edentulism. In all cases, a removable complete denture is an essential step in the treatment process, even if it is only a temporary stage in preparation for an implant-supported prosthesis. Dentists need to master the technique for fabricating immediate dentures so that their edentulous patients will not lose oral functions. Now that this technique is precisely outlined and described, it offers practitioners a dependable and clinically proven prosthetic option. Its benefits include preservation of anteroposterior basal bone, thus ensuring sufficient available bone for esthetic restoration with an implant-supported prosthesis.

Successive prosthetic treatments can lead patients who are approaching edentulism to develop habits and dysfunctional oral behavior (more or less iatrogenic in nature), which make them poor candidates for an implant-supported prosthesis immediately following extraction of their remaining teeth. Dentists will find, therefore, that the use of a temporary prosthesis whose therapeutic function is to maintain or re-establish "comfortable" function will have a beneficial effect on the overall success of treatment. Patients are more willing to accept ongoing treatment that protects their oral health when their prosthetic restorations maintain or re-establish both proper relationships between the jaws and good esthetics, as well as assist them in speaking and swallowing properly.

Summing up

The immediate complete denture has these advantages:

- From the outset, the prosthesis is functional. Thus, patients approaching the end of their treatment feel better able to adapt to their new situation in full confidence.
- Stability of the occlusal and vertical dimensions is ensured by precise registration of the maxillomandibular relationship.
- Use of custom impression techniques and precision placement of artificial teeth establish the mechanical equilibrium of the prosthesis.
- Biologic integrity of the bone and the mucosa is maintained. If extractions are well planned and executed with the aid of a surgical guide, resorption of the supporting tissues is kept to a minimum. Paradoxically, good surgical technique in removing teeth preserves bone!
- Esthetic goals are achieved by maintaining (or in some cases improving) the patient's appearance, which is especially important with young patients.

In this book, we describe the fabrication of an immediate complete denture, a technique that was presented for the first time in France in 1978 by Pierre Buchard, Georges Apap, Maurice Navarro, and Jean-Marie Rignon-Bret.

This approach, whose primary principles we retain here, has since been improved upon as described by Jean-Marie Rignon-Bret in a large number of articles and books (see Suggested Readings). In this book, we further develop innovations on these concepts.

We use a principal clinical case (whose illustrations are enclosed in a red border) to demonstrate precisely, step by step, the different stages of treatment. Alongside this presentation, we develop specific points based on what we encountered with other patients. Finally, in the last chapter, we describe the adaptations that must be made to deal with a variety of other clinical situations.

Clinical
Conditions

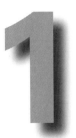

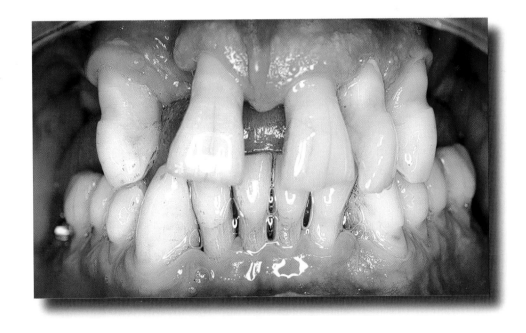

General Clinical Conditions

Use of an immediate complete denture in the maxilla requires that certain clinical conditions be met:

- All premolars and molars must be absent on both the right and left sides. The posterior regions that will support the denture must have stable osseous and mucosal tissues that are completely healed. Usually, a 3-month period is sufficient after posterior teeth have been extracted for healing to occur. Posterior alveolar ridges that are able to support the immediate denture facilitate the healing of the anterior maxilla following extraction of the remaining incisors and canines.
- The practitioner must ensure the stability and retention of the prosthesis by taking primary and secondary impressions.
- The practitioner should record the vertical relationship between the jaws using the proposed maxillary denture as a base line for the occlusal plane in which the mandibular teeth will eventually articulate. Thus, the mandibular plane of occlusion contributes to the functional mounting of the maxillary denture, which in turn contributes to the mounting of the anterior teeth on the articulator. This means that the opposing occlusal plane must be modified on the day the immediate denture is placed, just before surgery. While the denture is being constructed, the patient can get along without posterior teeth if the remaining teeth maintain a good maxillomandibular relationship. If not, a provisional denture should be fabricated.
- The practitioner must understand the physiology of the masticatory system.
- The esthetics of the denture should be established in advance in keeping with the patient's wishes.
- The practitioner must understand the patient's psychological needs during the transition period prior to placement of the new denture.
- The patient must be healthy enough to undergo the surgical procedures associated with tooth extraction and possible osseous surgery.
- The practitioner must understand the healing of the surgical sites and be able to predict the outcome of the necessary extractions.

Principal Clinical Case

The patient, who is in his forties, exhibits good facial balance at each level of his profile, with the firm and harmonious support of his upper lip (Fig 1-1). When occluded, the remaining teeth demonstrate a stable maxillomandibular relationship with a well-functioning vertical dimension, just as the contours of his face would suggest (Fig 1-2). When the patient smiles, the edges of the slightly extruded maxillary incisors can be seen in relation to the upper lip. The practitioner must take the extruded position of the maxillary dentition into account when the interincisal junction is established on the prosthesis (Fig 1-3).

The extent of resorption in the alveolar ridge is clearly visible in periapical and panoramic radiographs (Fig 1-4) and will be a determining factor in the preparation of the definitive working cast.

In the mandible, 12 natural teeth are still present (Figs 1-5 and 1-6). The second molars are missing, which will complicate the task of equilibrating the maxillary denture base during protrusive mandibular movements. The denture must be constructed so that there are bilateral balanced generalized contacts between the two arches during protrusive movements. The maxilla is edentulous in the posterior regions but still bears five anterior teeth, three incisors and the canines. The posterior maxillary regions are stable (Fig 1-7).

There are no pathological conditions that would contraindicate oral surgery.

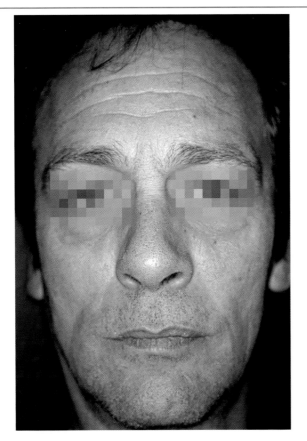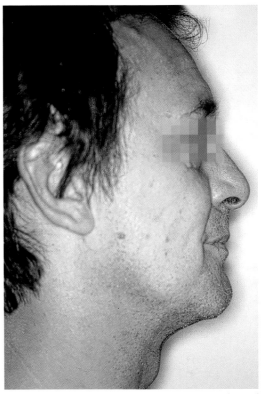

Figs 1-1a and 1-1b The patient's face in frontal *(a, left)* and profile *(b, right)* views.

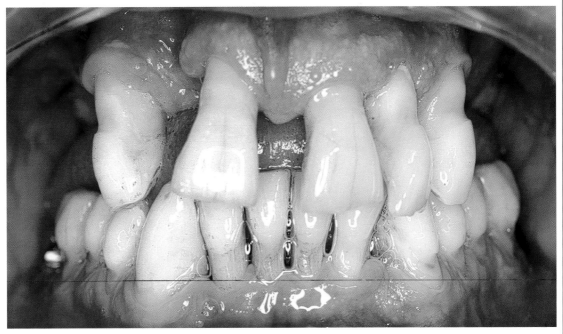

Fig 1-2 The remaining dentition in habitual occlusion.

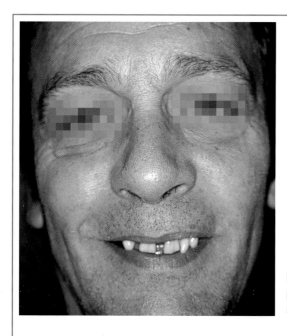

Fig 1-3 Smiling slightly, the patient reveals the position of his maxillary incisors and their relationship to the upper lip.

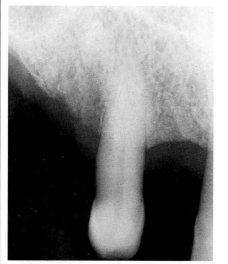
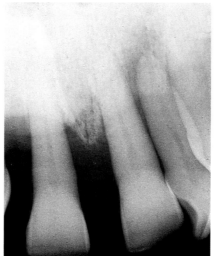
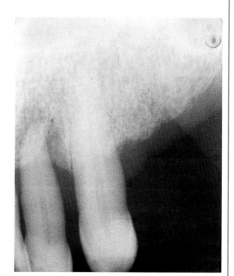

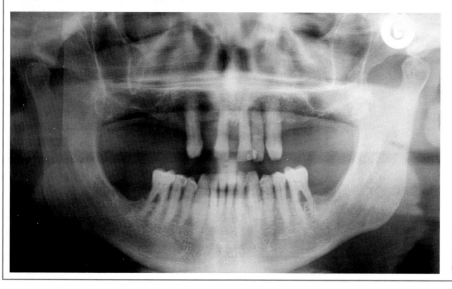

Figs 1-4a to 1-4d Periapical *(a to c, top)* and panoramic *(d, left)* radiographs indicate the extent of alveolar bone resorption.

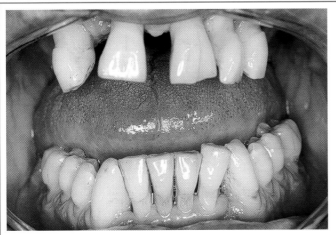

Fig 1-5 The opposing arch. The number and positioning of the teeth assure a unified occlusal unit. The second premolars and first molars, on both sides, represent the center of the prosthetic equilibrium.

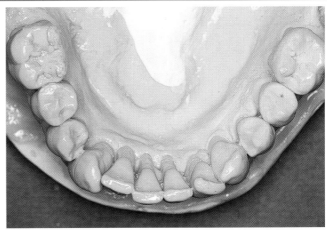

Fig 1-6 The working cast of the mandible.

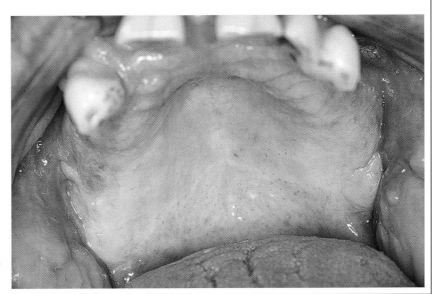

Fig 1-7 The edentulous posterior maxilla prior to impression taking.

Objective

The treatment objective is to construct a complete removable maxillary denture that is ready for placement immediately following extraction of the five remaining teeth. A surgical guide will be used to assist in the shaping of the alveolar ridges after tooth extraction has been completed. With the teeth in occlusion, the surgical guide will point out the best positioning for the denture base so that, when it is in place in the maxilla, the denture can assist the healing of mucosal and osseous tissues and keep the patient comfortable. In follow-up visits, the dentist can make any necessary adjustments to ensure the integration of the maxillary prosthesis with the stomatognathic system.

Impressions

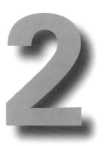

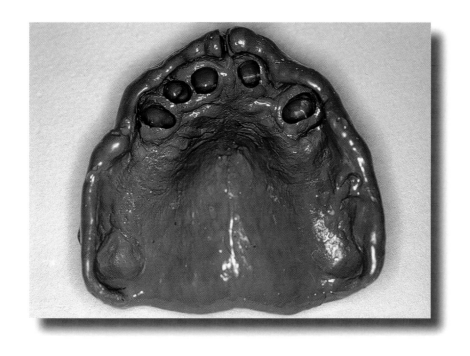

Primary Impressions

Objective
The goal in taking the primary impression is to obtain an accurate replica of both dentate and edentulous areas. The depth of the vestibular fold and the soft palate are also included in the primary impression, which should be taken with as little deformation of the soft tissues in the edentulous areas and as little displacement of the remaining teeth as possible.

The primary impression should be taken carefully. Any deficiencies will carry over to the custom impression tray constructed from the cast that is subsequently used to take the definitive impression.

> The practitioner should not accept an inaccurate impression even when the presence of residual teeth make achieving a truly satisfactory impression technically difficult.

Materials
– A nonperforated stock impression tray. This tray assures the best impression material placement.
– A 60-mL syringe with a large central barrel of the type used for parenteral feeding, and/or a wooden tongue depressor (Fig 2-1)
– Type 1 alginate

Step-by-Step Clinical Procedure
The chief problem practitioners encounter in taking the primary impression is difficulty removing it from the patient's mouth because of the presence of residual anterior teeth. Practitioners should anticipate this problem and select an impression tray larger than the dental arch. The tray can be further extended with wax as needed to accommodate individual morphology so that, for example, extruded anterior teeth will be fully covered (Fig 2-2). This procedure, however, is usually not necessary.

In taking the primary impression, practitioners should follow these steps:
1. Mix the alginate with ice-cold water in a water-powder ratio slightly lower than normal so that the consistency will be thicker and the material will have a longer setting time. After it is placed in the impression tray, it can easily be shaped roughly to conform to the anatomy of the arch (Fig 2-3).
2. Using a syringe or tongue depressor, place some of the alginate in the mucobuccal folds and on the soft palate, as well as around the remaining teeth and on the retromolar tuberosities before seating the filled tray (Fig 2-4).
3. Check the tray after placement in the mouth to be sure that it is centered and correctly positioned over the soft palate.
4. Ask the patient, who to this point has been sitting upright, to lower his or her head.

> While gently guiding the patient's head, check again to be certain that the anterior teeth are well situated in the anterior sector of the tray, at the same time guiding the patient's upper lip to lie comfortably around the tray.

5. Continue to hold both the tray and the patient's head until the impression material has set.
6. Finally, remove the tray, which is usually not difficult to do.

After checking the impression for quality, the practitioner should rinse it off, disinfect it, and pack it properly for shipping to the laboratory (Fig 2-5).

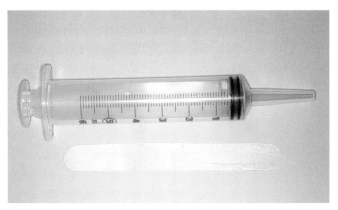

Fig 2-1 Large-barrel syringe and tongue depressor.

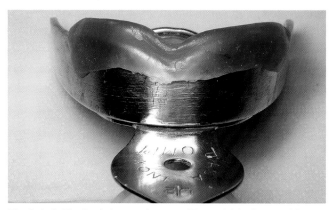

Fig 2-2 A Rim-Lock impression tray (Dentsply) built up with wax anteriorly.

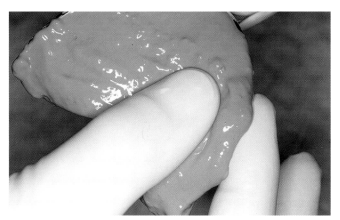

Fig 2-3 Roughly shaping the alginate.

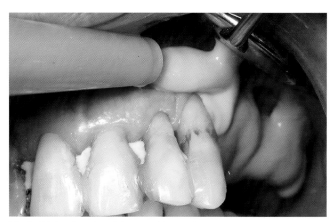

Fig 2-4 Injecting the alginate with a syringe.

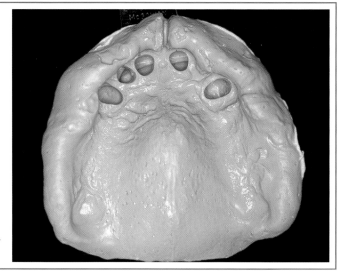

Fig 2-5 Primary alginate impression.

A few bubbles or a spot or two where the impression tray shows through do not render an impression unacceptable. Insufficiency on the ridge-supporting surfaces, in the depth of the mucobuccal fold, or in the palatal region is, however, sufficient reason to retake the impression.

Clinical Variations

The few remaining teeth in a prospective immediate denture patient are frequently so mobile and so widely separated from periodontal drift that practitioners often fear the teeth may be inadvertently extracted in the impression.

In such cases, the practitioner should:
- Fill the interdental spaces with a product such as nonpolymerized silicone, especially if the teeth have been supported by a temporary splint.
- Then, splint them more solidly with a temporary bonding material such as cyanoacrylate.
- Burnish some tinfoil over the teeth and marginal gingiva.

Trays with relief compartments designed for taking primary impressions in Kennedy Class 1 edentulous patients are available. Still, trays that fit the precise anatomic patterns of individual patients are hard to find because both the anterior and the posterior compartments of the tray must match the patient's anatomy.

Custom Impression Trays

Objective

The goal of taking the primary impression is to obtain working casts with which to fabricate custom impression trays for taking the secondary impression.

Materials

– Ordinary model plaster for pouring the cast.
– Auto- or photopolymerizable resin.
– Stent's impression compound.

Step-by-Step Laboratory Procedure

1. Preparing the primary impression. The cast should be poured as soon as possible. Once it has set, the cast should accurately represent all the elements sought in the impression—the teeth, the edentulous areas, the depth of the mucobuccal fold, and the soft palate (Figs 2-6 and 2-7). This cast should be trimmed so that its base is at least 1 cm thick, parallel to the Copperman plane, and angled in such a way that the mucobuccal fold on the cast can be easily accessed.

2. Outlining the borders of the custom impression tray. In edentulous areas, the borders of the impression tray should be located 1 to 1.5 mm above the depth of the mucobuccal fold and in the soft palate at the point where the folding of the palate can be visualized when the patient slowly pronounces a long "A" (Figs 2-8 and 2-9). The presence of teeth and undercuts in the anterior region makes it impossible to extend the tray as deeply as in posterior areas. Practitioners should trace the outline anteriorly along the greatest-bulge of tissue over which the tray will be inserted and withdrawn (Fig 2-10).

3. Making the custom impression tray. The remaining teeth and marginal gingiva are covered with a thin, 1-mm spacer sheet of wax that stops short of the outlined border to

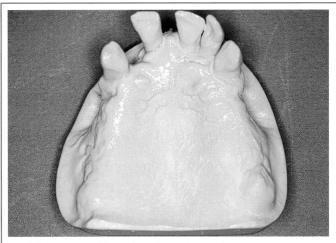

Fig 2-6 Cast poured from the primary impression.

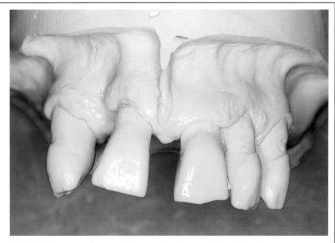

Fig 2-7 The anterior maxilla precisely reproduced in plaster.

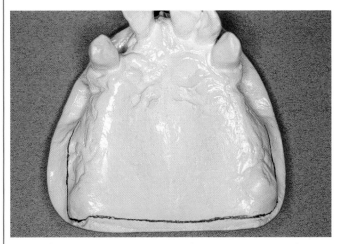

Fig 2-8 Outline of the posterior border for the custom impression tray.

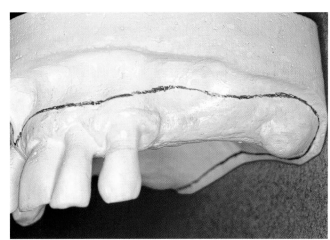

Fig 2-9 Outline of the lateral border for the custom impression tray.

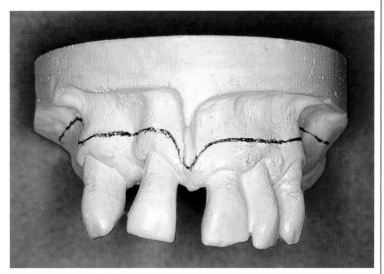

Fig 2-10 Outline of the anterior border for the custom impression tray.

which the custom tray will be adapted (Fig 2-11). The spacing provided by the wax creates a little room for the anterior part of the custom tray after polymerization, so that it can be removed smoothly (Fig 2-12).

After an isolating film is placed on the cast, the palatal basin of the tray is made with a sheet of resin of precalibrated thickness. When polymerization is complete, the practitioner trims the tray to match the borders as outlined (Fig 2-13).

Finally, the practitioner places occlusal rims of Stent's impression compound or resin on the edentulous ridge areas so that there will be adequate space for prosthetic teeth when the secondary impression is taken (Fig 2-14).

Clinical Variations

It is a good idea to make the anterior part of the custom tray detachable to eliminate the risk of fracturing the anterior teeth when the secondary impression is removed from the cast.

Therefore, the posterior part of the custom impression tray, which begins just distal to the wax covering the residual anterior teeth, is made first and covered with a light coat of petroleum jelly. When the resin has hardened, the anterior buccal segment is made and its fit to the posterior part is checked. The two parts of the impression tray, anterior and posterior, are joined by metallic brads that are heated before being plunged into the acrylic at the juncture of the two parts, but well away from the buccal areas that will need trimming. When the impression tray is used to take the secondary impression, the brads are cut and the anterior and posterior parts are removed separately (Fig 2-15).

If the maxillary anterior teeth have a marked labial inclination, it is sometimes a good idea to construct the custom tray without a separate anterior section so as not to interfere with lip support (Fig 2-16). Another technique is simply to detach the anterior section and use it as a separate tray, not coated with adhesive, that can be removed without disturbing the mobile, protruding incisors.

Alternatively, the practitioner can fashion an anterior window in the custom impression tray with the lower, supporting part of the segment left in place (Fig 2-17).

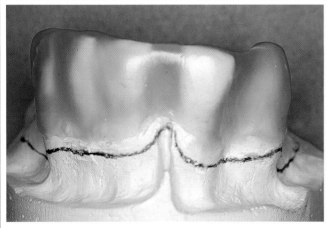 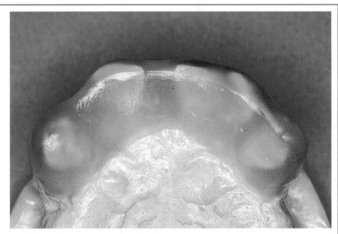

Figs 2-11a and 2-11b Spacing wax adapted to the remaining teeth: buccal *(a, left)* and palatal *(b, right)* views.

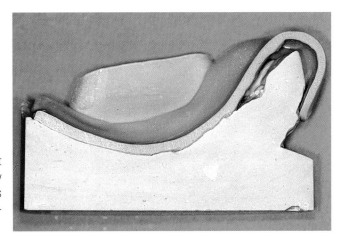

Fig 2-12 Cross section of the cast and the custom impression tray showing how the spacing wax has left a protective gap over the remaining anterior teeth.

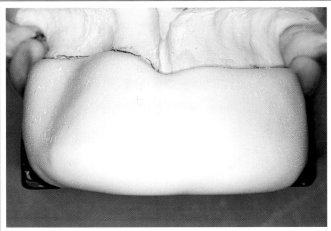

Fig 2-13 Frontal view of a custom impression tray that has been trimmed along the outline.

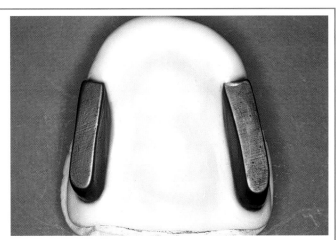

Fig 2-14 Custom impression tray with occlusal rims in the buccal areas where prosthetic teeth will later be inserted.

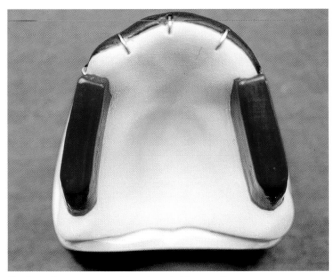

Fig 2-15 Custom tray with a detachable anterior component.

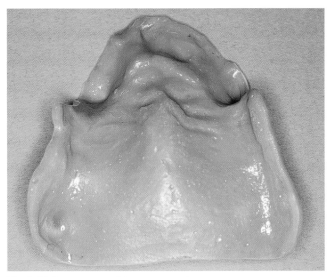

Fig 2-16 Custom tray without an anterior component.

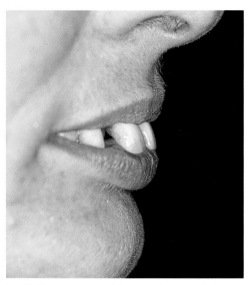

Fig 2-17a A patient with severely protruded maxillary anterior teeth.

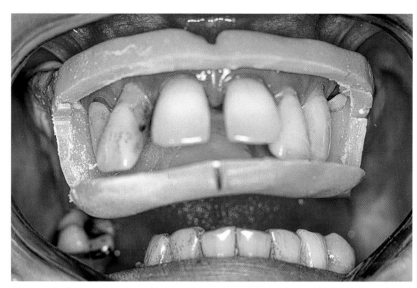

Fig 2-17b To accommodate the anterior teeth, a labial window has been cut in the custom tray, with the base of the tray left intact.

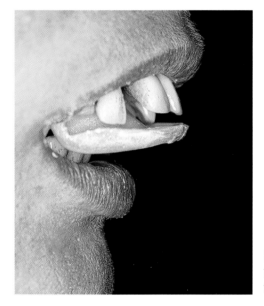

Fig 2-17c When positioned in the mouth, the custom tray interferes very little with the upper lip.

Secondary Impressions

Objective

In taking the secondary impression, the practitioner's goal is to obtain a cast that can be used to fabricate a complete denture with adequate support and retention. Therefore, the impression is extended as deeply and as widely as possible to register the supporting areas without the impression becoming too thick or having overhangs. In edentulous areas, practitioners can follow the standard technique for fabricating complete removable dentures, but in areas where teeth and possibly undercuts are present, determining the limits of the impression is more difficult.

This problem is exacerbated when mobile anterior teeth project so far forward that they interfere with normal functioning of the orbicular lip musculature.

Materials Typically Used in Complete Denture Fabrication

– Custom impression tray.

> The labial border of the anterior part of the custom tray is located along the maximum convexity of the alveolar process if residual teeth are present.

In fact, if it were to be placed any deeper, it would be too far from the fibromucosa of the mucobuccal fold. Such overcontouring would make accurate determination of the anterior border of the complete denture difficult if not impossible.

– Impression compound (soft green, Kerr) for registering the functional borders of the edentulous sectors and recording the juncture of the soft and hard palates.
– Low-viscosity polysulfide (light-bodied Permlastic, Kerr) for the details around the remaining dentition. This material does not become too rigid after polymerization, which makes it easier to remove from the mouth and minimizes the risk of inadvertent extraction of overly mobile teeth.
– Alternatively, practitioners may choose polyethers, such as light- or heavy-body Permadyne (3M/ESPE) or Impregum F (3M/ESPE), for every part of the impression. Polyethers are always used in the anterior portion when the custom tray consists of two detachable parts.

Step-by-Step Clinical Procedure

1. The practitioner tries the custom impression tray in the patient's mouth and eliminates any overhangs and excessively thick areas on the lateral and posterior borders, using the standard techniques for removable complete dentures.
2. The practitioner registers the functional limits for the proposed prosthesis in the edentulous areas as well as at the vibrating line using either Kerr's soft green impression compound (Fig 2-18) or a polyether for this purpose (Figs 2-19a to 2-19f). With the impression tray in place, the practitioner asks the patient to:
   • Move the mandible to the right, then to left, and suck in the cheeks to mold the material in the lateral area.
   • Say "ah" and hold the sound for the registration of the vibrating line.

The sequence of steps followed in taking the impression of the posterior portion in the custom tray differs from the sequence followed in conventional technique for making complete dentures. For the immediate complete denture, the practitioner makes an impression

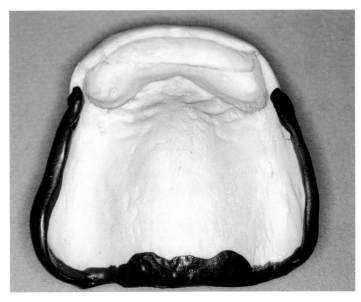

Fig 2-18 Registration of the lateral borders and the vibrating line with Kerr's soft green impression compound.

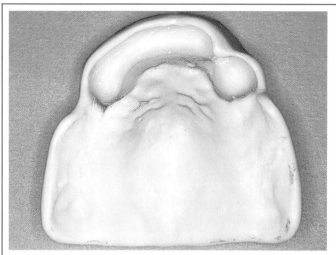

Fig 2-19a Registration of the lateral borders of the custom tray. The practitioner has trimmed the tray following standard procedure for making a complete denture.

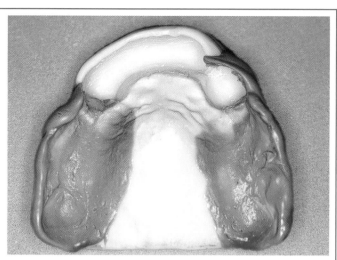

Fig 2-19b First registration, done with Permadyne.

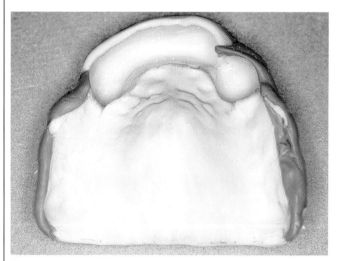

Fig 2-19c Appearance after removal of excess or overhanging material.

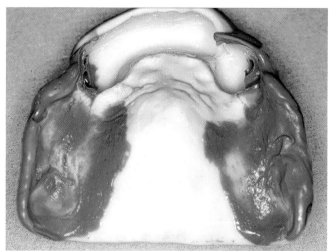

Fig 2-19d A second registration is done with Impregum.

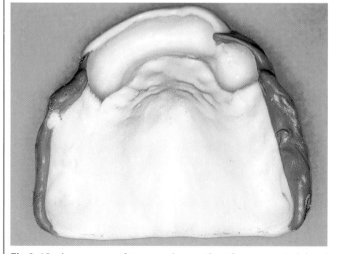

Fig 2-19e Appearance after second correction of excess material and overhangs.

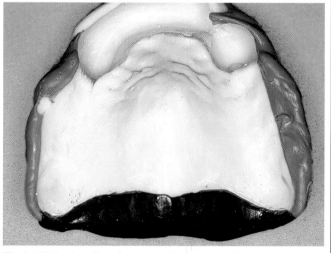

Fig 2-19f Kerr's soft green impression compound used to obtain an impression of the vibrating line.

of the posterior region before registering the anterior region.

3. The next step is to set up the hinged anterior sector (Fig 2-20).

Polyether impression materials can be gently molded into shape even if they are not supported by the walls of an impression tray, and so readily show areas of excessive thickness or overhangs.

The impression of the hinged anterior sector is made with Permadyne placed along the edges of the custom tray. The material can be formed into shape by finger molding with moistened gloves or injected directly into the patient's mouth with a Ramitec-type syringe (3M Dental) (Fig 2-21).

The patient is then asked to:
• Suck in the cheeks.
• Smile, pulling back the lips while doing so.
• Purse the lips and advance them as though kissing someone.

After polymerization is completed, the practitioner examines the impression, eliminates excess material, and take another impression with a material of lower viscosity, such as Impregnum F (Figs 2-22 and 2-23).

4. If the juncture with the anterior segment appears satisfactory, shows no break in continuity with the lateral sectors, and causes no esthetic deformation, the practitioner can proceed to the final relining stage. In this stage the inner curve of the arches, the anterior recess for the teeth, and the borders are coated with Permlastic, a low-viscosity polysulfide, and the custom tray is reinserted into the patient's mouth. The practitioner holds the tray firmly in place with high finger pressure applied to the areas of the second premolars and first molars, which will be the center of equilibrium of the future prosthesis. The patient, still seated upright, is asked to repeat several times the lip and cheek molding procedures as before.

To be considered satisfactory, the impression should have no insufficiencies in the anterior region of the remaining teeth or on the ridge-bearing surfaces, nor should there be any deformations resulting from excessive thickness or thinness in the border regions (Figs 2-24 and 2-25).

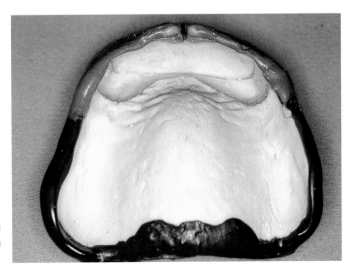

Fig 2-20 The lateral and post dam impressions were made with soft green impression compound, and the anterior impression was made with polyethers.

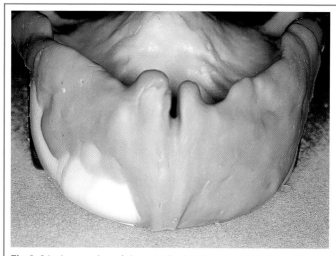

Fig 2-21a Impression of the anterior border made with Permadyne.

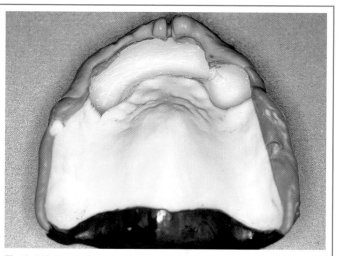

Fig 2-21b Internal excess is removed.

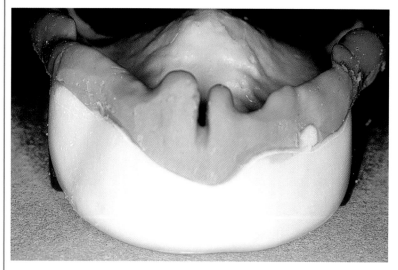

Fig 2-21c Excess border impression material in the buccal area is trimmed away.

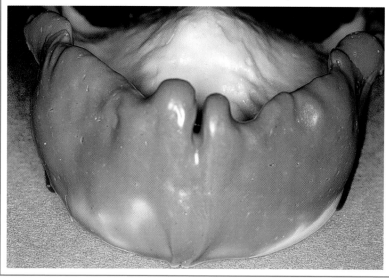

Fig 2-22 A final impression is made with Impregnum F.

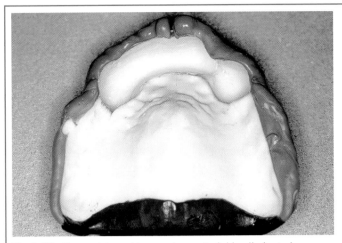

Fig 2-23a Excess internal impression material is eliminated.

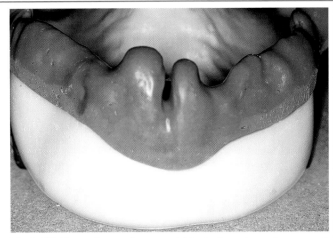

Fig 2-23b Excess impression material in the buccal area is removed.

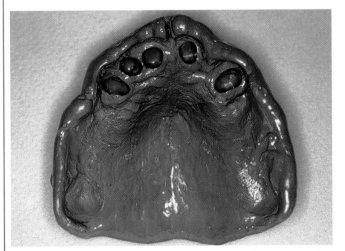

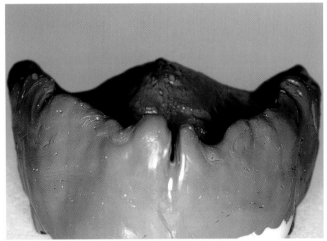

Figs 2-24a and 2-24b Final impression made with low-viscosity Permlastic: an internal view *(a, left)* and labial view *(b, right)*.

Fig 2-25 The lateral and the posterior dam impressions have been made with Kerr's soft green impression compound, the anterior portion with polyethers. The relining was accomplished with low-viscosity polysulfide.

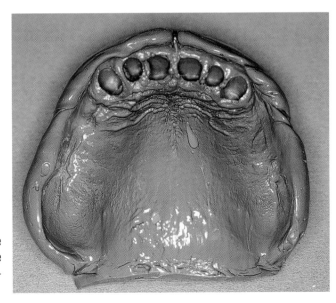

Clinical Variations

If the remaining teeth are very mobile, the practitioner should be careful to follow the procedures already described to avoid inadvertent extraction. However, blocking out interdental spaces and/or applying a layer of tin foil to the crowns may obliterate details.

Teeth that are severely inclined labially are frequently problematic. They can interfere with the activity of the orbicularis musculature, making it difficult for the practitioner to obtain a good impression (Fig 2-26). If the resin layer is too thick in this area it can exacerbate the problem and falsify the registration by thickening and enlarging the anterior impression. In such cases, the polyethers are rigid enough after polymerization to permit a final impression to be made using a custom impression tray that has no anterior component.

To take secondary impressions of highly mobile remaining teeth, the practitioner first makes the posterior impression, checks it, and reseats the tray (Fig 2-27). To complete the anterior segment, the practitioner injects polyether around the teeth with a Ramitec-type syringe (Fig 2-28). This secondary impression should be removed carefully, in the direction of the long axis of the fragile anterior teeth.

When the custom tray has been designed with a window in the anterior labial portion, the practitioner takes an impression of the "soft joint" sector first, then takes the relining impression of the posterior support surfaces. Only then is the impression material injected into the anterior segment (Figs 2-29 and 2-30).

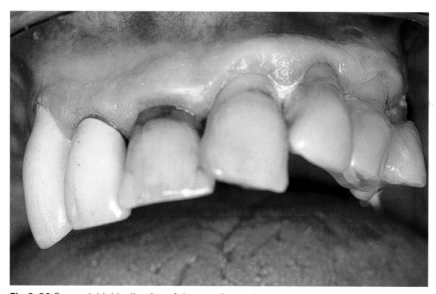

Fig 2-26 Severe labial inclination of the anterior teeth.

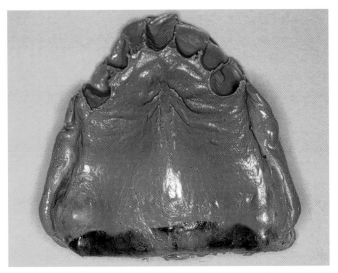

Fig 2-27 Impression taken of the posterior sector as a first step.

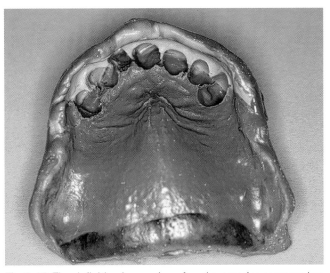

Fig 2-28 The definitive impression after the anterior segment has been added.

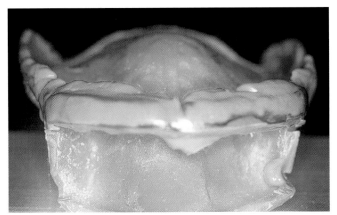
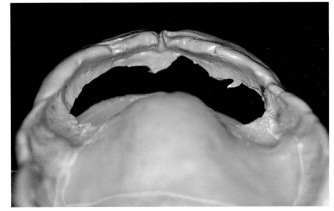

Figs 2-29a and 2-29b Custom tray with a window in the anterior "soft joint" sector: labial view *(a, left)* and view from the palate onto the inner surface. *(b, right).*

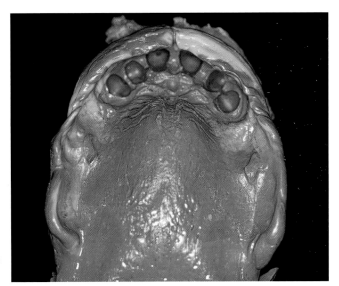

Fig 2-30 A relining impression made with Permadyne, the material of choice when the remaining teeth are not mobile.

Maxillomandibular Relationship

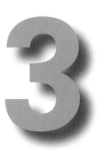

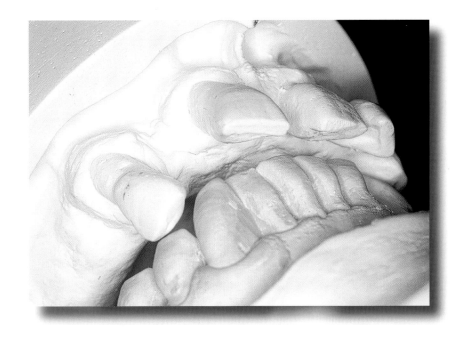

Denture Bases

Objective

The definitive impression is used to pour a master cast on which the prosthesis will be fabricated. The occlusal base, which also serves as a transfer base, is first used to mount the maxillary cast on an articulator, and then for mounting the mandibular cast on the lower part of the articulator in the appropriate maxillomandibular relationship as registered clinically.

Materials

– Model plaster (type II or III) specifically designed for full denture construction. Because immediate complete dentures require a modifiable cast, hard, type IV high-strength dental stone cannot be used.
– Trubase (Dentsply) or an impression tray resin.
– Stent's impression compound.
– Zinc oxide-eugenol impression paste.

Step-by-Step Laboratory Procedure

1. Approach to the impression and master cast. The definitive impression is boxed to preserve the functional limits registered along its periphery (Fig 3-1). In edentulous areas the framework of the wax box is positioned at the level of the greatest contour bulge. In anterior, dentate areas it is positioned 2 to 3 mm from the depth of the mucobuccal fold.

> The impression should be removed from the cast along a vector that will not risk fracturing the plaster teeth.

If the practitioner has taken a separate detachable impression of the anterior segment, that should be removed first (Fig 3-2). Otherwise, a generous anterior window should be cut away (Fig 3-3).

The master cast (Fig 3-4) should have a base that is poured or trimmed parallel to the Copperman plane and is at least 1 cm thick.

2. The denture base. Any posterior undercuts should be filled in with silicone before the cast is prepared with petroleum jelly or another isolating film. Trubase or a resin is then applied to the palatal vault, denture ridges, and into the mucobuccal fold on the cast, with the necks of the anterior teeth marking the anterior limit. Occlusal rims are placed on the right and left edentulous posterior ridges and should be at least 2 mm higher than the remaining teeth (Figs 3-5 and 3-6). In order to ensure that the denture base will remain in place during registrations, zinc oxide eugenol paste can be used to stabilize the occlusal base on the isolated cast.

Clinical Variations

The denture base can be made more retentive by the addition of two clasps.

When remaining teeth are extremely abraded, they can be overlaid with a silicone strip to extend the anterior part of the denture base. The silicone strip is placed over the palatal and occlusal surfaces of the anterior teeth aligned with the occlusal base and helps establishe the midincisal point (see next chapter).

This silicone strip can be used in other clinical situations to reference a future prosthetic midincisal point (Fig 3-7).

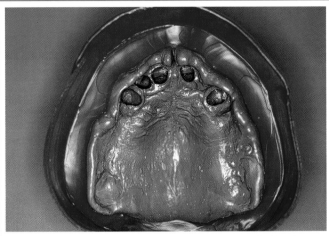

Fig 3-1 Boxing of an impression to preserve the recorded borders.

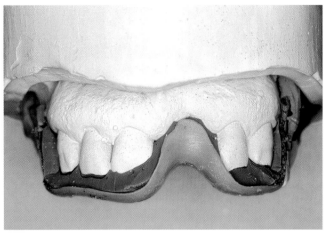

Fig 3-2 The poured cast removed from the impression. There are no fractured teeth in the cast, thanks to the incorporation of an anterior detachable window.

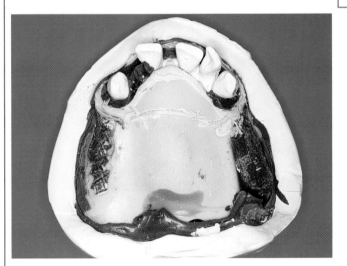

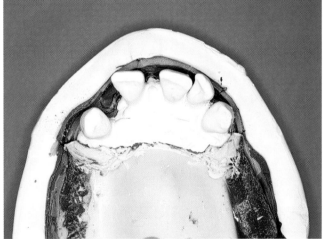

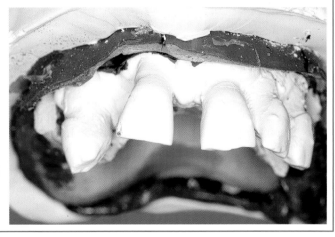

Figs 3-3a to 3-3c Separation of the cast *(a, top left; b, top right)*. In c *(right)*, the final impression has been cut away to reveal the cast of the remaining teeth.

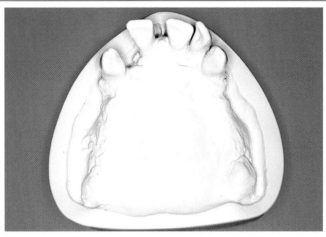
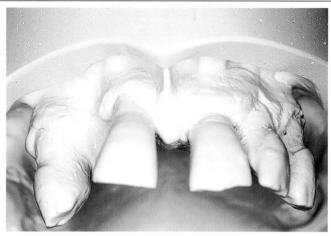

Figs 3-4a and 3-4b Master cast: occlusal view *(a, left)* and a detail of the anterior dentition *(b, right)*. The anatomic details of the impression have been faithfully rendered in stone.

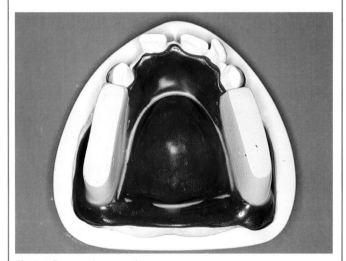

Fig 3-5 Denture base on the cast.

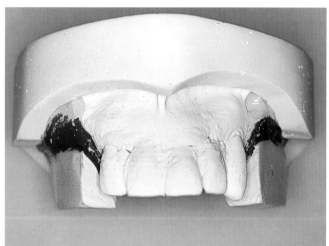

Fig 3-6 The occlusal rims are 2 mm higher than the remaining natural teeth.

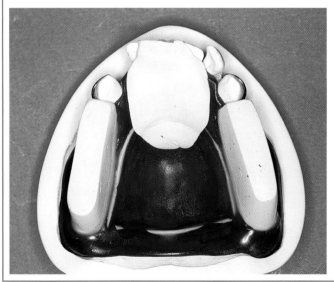

Fig 3-7 The anterior sector of the denture base is extended with a strip of silicone that will help establish the midincisal point.

The Midincisal Point

Objectives

Establishing the midincisal point can be a simple step or one of the most complicated steps of fabricating a denture. Its goals are:

- Mounting the maxillary cast on the articulator
- Preserving or restoring the anterior esthetics

If the remaining teeth are extruded, the transfer plane of the cast will be situated lower than normal. Vertical adjustment to the articulator restores the midincisal point within the articulator's geometric scope. The midincisal point of the prosthesis is established clinically based on the patient's natural midincisal point. It must be transferred precisely using an anterior bite index of the patient's preoperative situation designed for an esthetic mounting of the cast.

Assessment

Clinically, it is frequently very difficult to validate the midincisal point of the denture. It must be deduced from the natural midincisal point. In trying to locate the midincisal point, the clinician may encounter five different situations.

The natural midincisal point can be:

- Preserved and is easily transferred to the articulator.
- Drifted to one side and needs only to be recentered using the facial midline as a guide.
- Displaced upward because of severe abrasion to the remaining teeth (Fig 3-8). The clinician must construct a silicone index that extends to the anterior dentition along the transfer plane, thus establishing a new anterior limit as well as the midincisal point of the prosthesis (Fig 3-9).
- Displaced downward because of Class II malocclusions, which results in an excessively gummy smile. This interference with the transfer plane requires the cast to be remounted.
- Displaced forward, which is often accompanied by an additional upward displacement. This is a result of protruded maxillary teeth (Fig 3-10).

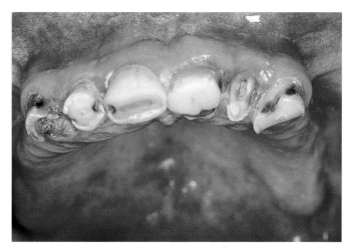

Fig 3-8 Severely abraded teeth.

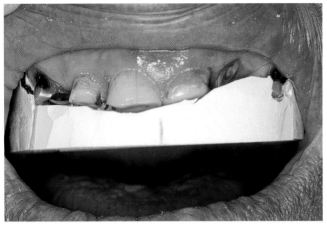

Fig 3-9a The midincisal point is established with a silicone index.

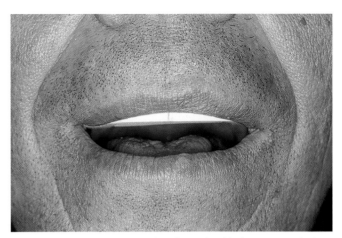

Fig 3-9b Esthetic positioning is adjusted, with the same technique used in the traditional fabrication of complete dentures.

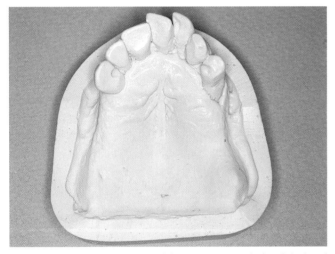

Fig 3-10a The anterior teeth on this cast are protruded and deviated laterally.

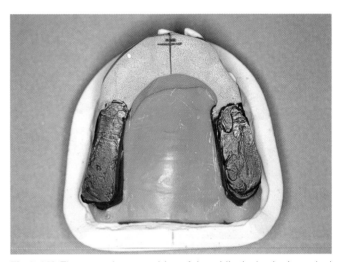

Fig 3-10b The approximate position of the midincisal point is marked on the occlusal surface of the silicone index.

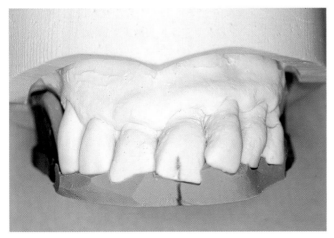

Fig 3-10c The midincisal point is indicated on the labial surface of the silicone index.

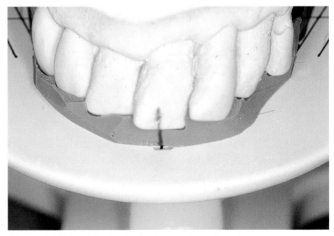

Fig 3-10d The midincisal point is transferred to the cast.

Note: The presence of a secondary diastema is a frequent indicator of the latter type of midincisal point displacement. However, it is difficult to know how much the midincisal point should be repositioned. It is, moreover, impossible to verify.

> In the majority of cases, the midincisal point is displaced in any spatial direction. The clinician must therefore rely on clinical experience and skill to establish the midincisal point for the prosthesis.

In extreme cases, a silicone index must be placed against the palatal surfaces of anterior teeth in harmony with the denture base (see Figs 3-10b and 3-10c). The position of the mandibular dentition, particularly any opposing anterior teeth, constitutes a valuable reference for positioning the maxillary denture base. However, the clinician must make allowance for factors that compromise the maxillomandibular relationships, such as severe erosion or drifting.

Step-by-Step Clinical Procedure
In some cases, the clinician has only to trace the midincisal point in the mouth and transfer it to the cast. For many patients, however, the clinician has to rely on the use of silicone indices (Figs 3-9 to 3-12).

1. The lateral occlusal blocks are paralleled to the transfer plane (parallel to the interpupillary line and Camper's plane) using a Fox occlusal plane guide. This plane must always pass beyond the incisal edges of the remaining teeth.
2. A silicone block is placed on the transfer base distal to the incisors and, using the Fox plane guide, moved into contact with the lateral blocks before polymerization.
3. Following polymerization, the clinician can use the silicone index to set the midincisal point (see Fig 3-11b).
   The silicone index provides:
   • effective management of the esthetic support for the upper lip, both at rest and in a smile.
   • simple registration of the midincisal point in keeping with the clinical situation (see Fig 3-12).
4. The maxillary cast should be placed on the transfer table of the articulator in accordance with the newly established midincisal point and the indicator cross traced on the table (see Fig 3-10d).

> The presence of extruded teeth sometimes requires a transfer plane that is lower than its exact position. The discrepancy can be compensated by a temporary raising of the articulator rod. Once it has been fixed, the cast is returned to its normal position.

Clinical Variations
These clinical variations depend on the position of the remaining anterior teeth and the clinician's goal for the final esthetic. When a patient presents with at least one edentulous ridge, an "esthetic try-in" will provide some idea of the final result.

After the denture base has been adjusted, the practitioner mounts the maxillary cast on the articulator using the transfer table prior to registration of the maxillomandibular relationships. In most cases involving remaining antagonistic teeth, markings on the maxillary occlusal rim are erased by bite marks made by the mandibular dentition.

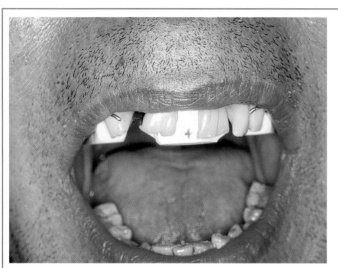

Fig 3-11a Determining the midincisal point of the denture.

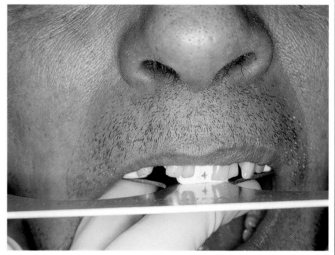

Fig 3-11b Verification of the transfer plane (parallel to Camper's base plane) with a Fox occlusal plane guide.

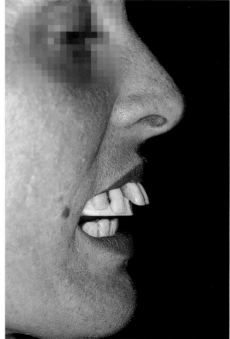

Fig 3-12a The midincisal point has been moved distally and lowered.

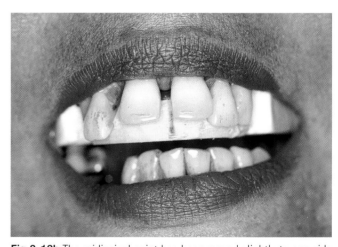

Fig 3-12b The midincisal point has been moved slightly to one side and lowered.

Registering the Maxillomandibular Relationship

Objectives

The mandible is positioned with respect to the maxilla to ensure maximal intercuspation on the prosthesis. The registration permits an evaluation of the vertical dimension and of the denture's balanced, centered, and symmetric position (horizontal and frontal dimensions).

Materials

– Maxillary denture base. After fulfilling the role of a transfer base, the denture base is placed on the articulator as an occlusal base.
– Mandibular denture base. Depending on how many mandibular teeth are missing, the dentist may have to use a mandibular occlusal base.

If feasible, the clinician should attempt to establish similar contacts between the jaws, with, for example, a maxillary occlusal rim against a mandibular occlusal rim or mandibular teeth. The clinician must position the arches in such a way that they will have sufficient internal support and support each other in occlusion.

Step-by-Step Laboratory Procedure

1. During setup, the mandibular teeth must be prevented from coming in contact with any remaining maxillary teeth. Such contacts might cause instability.

When the patient's vertical dimension of occlusion (VDO) has decreased, there is no risk of instability because the VDO for the prosthesis will necessarily exceed the actual VDO.

2. However, when the VDO has increased, the clinician may have to register in a slightly increased vertical dimension than the VDO, to avoid tooth-to-tooth contact (Figs 3-13 and 3-14).

3. By adjusting the articulator's vertical guide pin the practitioner will have no difficulty in restoring the correct vertical dimension.

4. When relations between occlusal rim and teeth need to be registered, Kerr's paste or wax can be used to record reference indentations, though they must eventually be re-indexed using zinc oxide-eugenol oxide paste (Fig 3-15).

5. During mandibular jaw movements, the clinician should guide the patient's mandible to avoid abnormal temporomandibular joint activity. If there is a mandibular occlusal base, the clinician can exert gentle bilateral posterior pressure. If there are remaining mandibular teeth, the clinician should provide directional guidance from the chin or by using the Dawson maneuver.

The patient should be instructed to raise his or her tongue back against the palate to encourage properposterior positioning of the mandible.

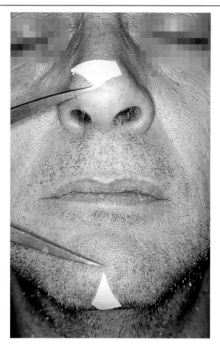

Fig 3-13 Determining the vertical dimension of registration (VDR), which is greater than the VDO.

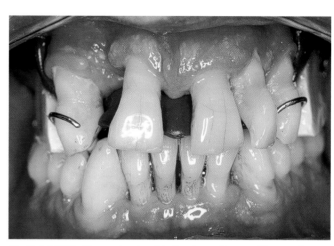

Fig 3-14 With the occlusal guide in place, the maxillary and mandibular anterior teeth are not in contact with each other.

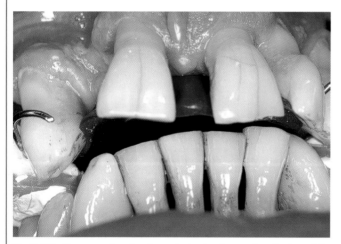

Fig 3-15a Close-up showing the anterior teeth out of occlusion while the practitioner records the VDR.

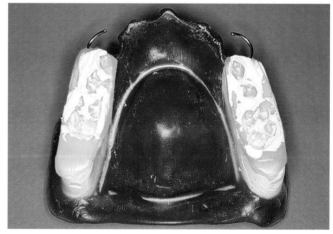

Fig 3-15b Zinc oxide eugenol paste has been applied to the mandibular occlusal rims. Before registering the maxillomandibular relationship, the clinician will mount the maxillary cast on the articulator.

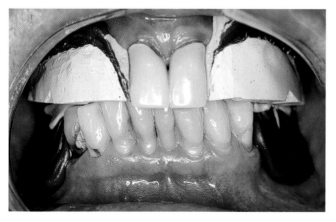

Fig 3-16 Registration of the maxillomandibular relationship of the maxillary and mandibular occlusal bases (the mandible represents a Kennedy Class I situation).

Clinical Variations

The desired vertical dimension for the prosthesis can be attained by reducing the occlusal rims. Reduction occurs first on those in the mandibular arch. If, however, mandibular teeth are present, the occlusal rims must be reduced on the maxillary cast, which is already mounted on the articulator. The adjustment continues until the VDR is reached.

At this stage, the relationship between the opposing occlusal rims is established via a system of interlacing markers. The maxillomandibular relationship is registered in wax (Kerr) using the RW Tench method, which is usually applied to conventional removable complete dentures (see Fig 3-16). Care must be taken to keep the occlusal rims from softening, which could compromise the vertical dimension stability. When the registration is taken, the practitioner should ask the patient to slowly close, stopping just before feeling any hard or resistant contact.

When the mandible represents a Kennedy Class II situation, contacts on each side of the dental arch are of a different nature. For patients who are completely edentulous or have a mandible with a Kennedy Class IV situation, no contact should be allowed between anterior teeth and the occlusal rims.

In every situation, the clinician should endeavor to set up conditions where both arches support each other. Finally, in cases of remaining posterior teeth in the mandible, the maxillary cast should be mounted on the articulator before the maxillomandibular relationship is registered.

Selecting Teeth

Objectives

Choosing and arranging artificial teeth constitute crucial elements in the preservation or, even, the improvement of esthetics. Moreover, the esthetic results are essential to the patient's acceptance of the prosthetic treatment. Traditionally, the clinician takes four factors into account—form, size, color, and material—when selecting artificial teeth.

Materials
– Form guides
– Shade guides
– Examples of prosthetic teeth

> Remaining anterior teeth can serve as an invaluable reference for the selection of artificial teeth. Nevertheless, the clinician must take into account modifications due to time and wear (eg, fissures, fractures, erosion, discoloration, and restorations).

Depending on the esthetic goals of the patient and practitioner, artificial teeth can be selected by:

- choosing artificial teeth that most closely resemble the original teeth and making modifications to mimic such characteristics as grinding and discoloration
- applying conventional protocol of complete denture prosthetics and selecting teeth that fit nicely with the natural teeth in size, form, and shade.

Step-by-Step Clinical Procedure
1. Ceramic teeth are usually selected for dentures. Depending on the preference for shade or form, practitioners begin their selection by examining shade or form guides (Fig 3-17).

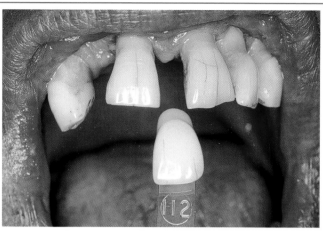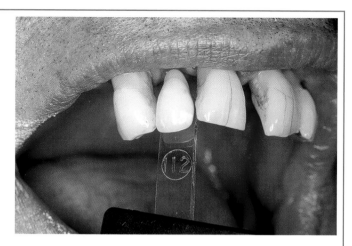

Figs 3-17a and 3-17b Selecting the shade of artificial teeth.

2. Once a preliminary decision has been made, the practitioner proceeds to narrow the selection by picking:
   • the best form available in the preferred shade
   • the best shade available in the preferred form
3. The size of the artificial teeth should match as close as possible to the dimensions of the patient's natural teeth before they were subjected to wear and tear.

Clinical Variations

Most patients want prosthetic teeth for a complete denture to improve on the arrangement as well as the appearance of their remaining natural teeth. This will frequently lead patients to want prosthetic teeth that are whiter and newer looking teeth than their natural dentition. The clinician must resist pressure to construct dentures whose whiteness and regularity proclaim artificiality.

If a patient presents old photographs of what his or her natural teeth, particularly those prior to restoration with fixed prostheses, the clinician can use this data during tooth selection but must adjust the final selection to correspond to the patient's current age.

Mounting the Casts on the Articulator

Objectives

Mounting casts on the articulator requires the clinician to stay within the "geometry" of the articulator while preserving the maxillomandibular relationship in the mouth.

Materials

– A dental articulator that fulfills basic requirements for the prosthetic concept to be applied
– Transfer and the denture bases

By using the incisal guide pin, the practitioner can adjust the midincisal point and variations of VDO.

Step-by-Step Clinical Procedure

1. The clinician positions the maxillary cast by superimposing its anteroposterior midline with the appropriate articulator axis and matching its marked midincisal point to the markings on the transfer table of the articulator (Fig 3-18).

   If the transfer plane is set lower than the determined midincisal point, the incisal guide pin can be raised to the extent of that gap and a third more, because the articulator guide pin is located anterior to the patient's midincisal point (Fig 3-19). This technique ensures that the midincisal point will line up correctly with the "geometry" of the articulator after the transfer table has been removed and the incisal guide pin reset at zero.

2. The opposing mandibular cast is oriented in the articulator at the proper VDR, which may be equal to or greater than the VDO (Fig 3-20).

   In cases where the VDR is greater than the VDO, the operator raises the incisal guide pin, which opens the articulator by the amount of the discrepancy plus one third to compensate for the difference between the patient and articulator. Once the teeth on the master cast are removed in keeping with extractions accomplished in the mouth, the incisal guide pin can be reset to zero, thus resetting the articulator to the correct VDO.

Clinical Variations

The outlined procedures cover the possible variation due to tooth loss in the maxilla or mandible.

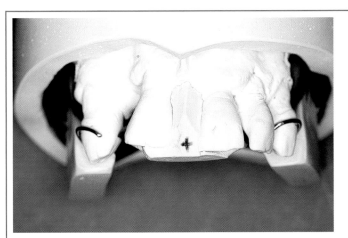
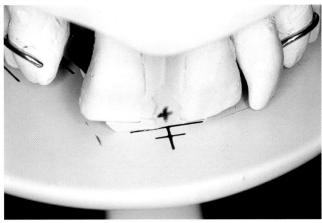

Figs 3-18a and 3-18b Transfer of the maxillary cast to the articulator. With the occlusal guide in place, the operator positions the cast on the transfer table.

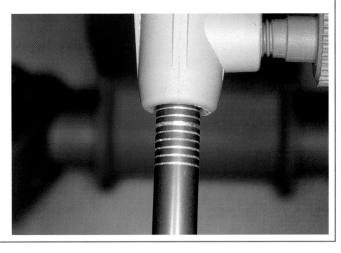

Fig 3-19 The incisal guide pin records the corrected vertical position of the prosthetic midincisal point.

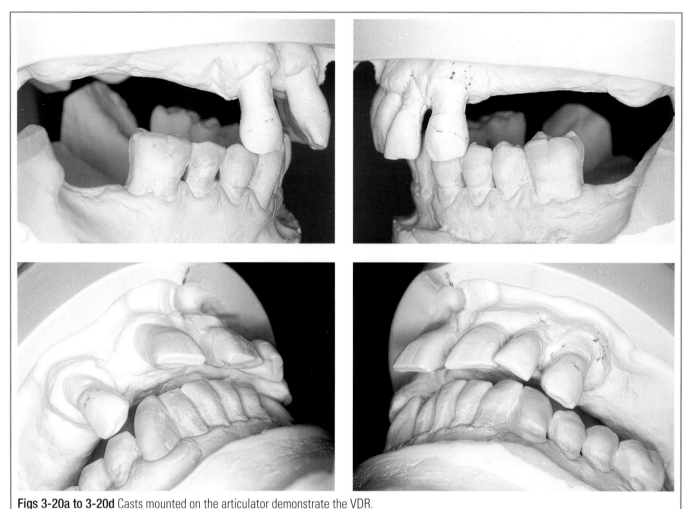

Figs 3-20a to 3-20d Casts mounted on the articulator demonstrate the VDR.

Waxed Dentures

Objectives
The practitioner can verify the planned prosthetic maxillomandibular relationship with the actual intraoral situation.

Materials
– Maxillary waxed denture incorporating posterior ceramic teeth of the desired shade with cusps angulated to articulate correctly with the mandibular dentition (Fig 3-21).
– If needed, mandibular waxed denture with artificial teeth installed.

Step-by-Step Laboratory Procedure
1. Softened wax is poured onto the edentulous areas on the cast.
2. Posterior artificial teeth are placed in softened wax at a height in accord with the predetermined VDR. No adjustment to teeth is made.
3. The wax mock-up is mounted with the remaining anterior dentition in place (see next chapter).

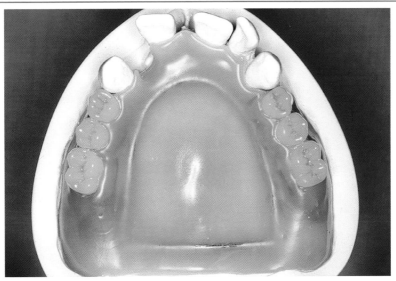

Fig 3-21a Maxillary wax mock-up demonstrating provisional positioning of the posterior ceramic teeth.

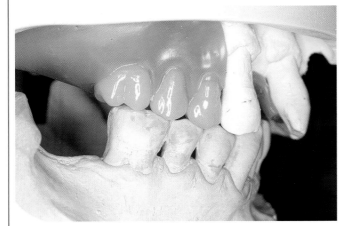 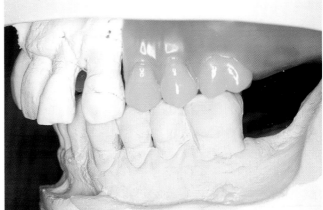

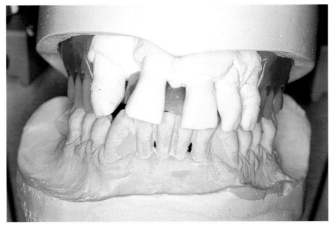

Figs 3-21b to 3-21d Lateral *(b and c, middle)* and frontal *(d)* views of the mock-up, provisionally mounted on the articulator at the VDR.

Clinical Variations

The practitioner can omit the waxed-denture stage for the posterior sector and proceed directly to the definitive arrangement of posterior teeth if:
- The VDR corresponds to the clinical VDO
- The setup of the anterior dentition anticipates no adjustment of the midincisal point and teeth positioning
- The opposing mandibular teeth require no major prosthetic restoration.

However, a posterior waxed denture allows the practitioner to verify that function and esthetics of the mock up are in harmonic agreement and to present the proposed arrangement to the patient before proceeding to the definitive arrangement.

In this case, the following procedure is proposed:

1. An impression is taken of the master cast with the wax mock-up from which a new plaster cast can be poured (Fig 3-22)
2. After the new cast is mounted on the articulator, the teeth are ground to articulate properly with the teeth on the mandibular cast.
3. The anterior teeth are removed for the buildup of a waxed denture in the esthetic zone (see next chapter) (Fig 3-23).

Therefore two casts are at the disposal of the practitioner, one demonstrating the posterior mock-up with the remaining anterior dentition and another with the proposed posterior

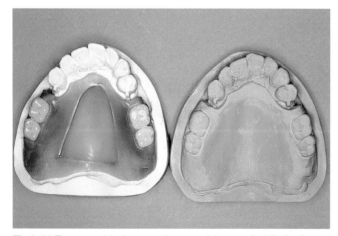

Fig 3-22 The cast with the posterior waxed denture *(left)* is duplicated to create a new plaster cast *(right)*.

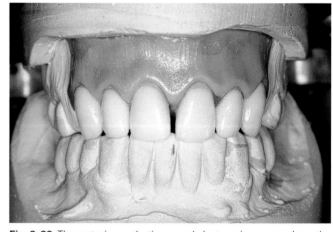

Fig 3-23 The anterior esthetic waxed denture is prepared on the modified new cast.

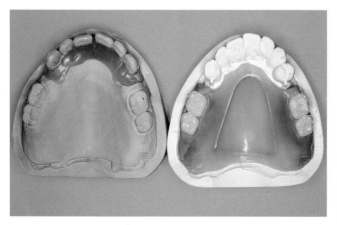

Fig 3-24 The modified duplicate cast with the removable anterior waxed denture *(left)* and the cast with the posterior waxed denture *(right)*.

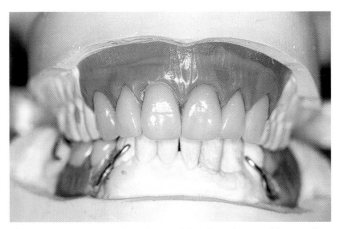 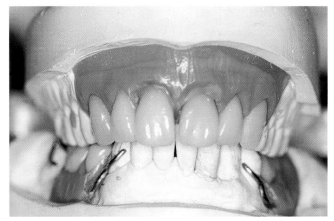

Figs 3-25a and 3-25b Anterior provisional mock-ups without a diastema *(a, left)* and with a slight midline diastema *(b, right).*

dentition and the anterior esthetic mock-up. Once the patient has approved the anterior esthetic waxed denture, it can be moved to the cast with the posterior waxed denture (Fig 3-24). In the present clinical case, the practitioner presents two esthetic options to the patient to decide the fate of an existing diastema between the central incisors (Fig 3-25).

Verifying the Maxillomandibular Relationship

Objectives
The relationship between the casts mounted on the articulator in maximum intercuspation must have a VDR that corresponds to the patient's VDR. If the practitioner finds a difference, a new vertical dimension must be registered, following the Tench method. At this stage, the clinician can also confirm the shade of the prosthetic teeth to the remaining dentition.

Materials
– Maxillary waxed denture.
– If needed, mandibular waxed denture.
– If a Tench rearticulation is needed, either wax and a sheet of silver foil or impression compound can be used.

Step-by-Step Clinical Procedure

1. The maxillary posterior waxed denture and, if needed, as well as the mandibular waxed denture are checked in the mouth. The practitioner guides the patient's jaw movements as was done for the registration of the maxillomandibular relationship (Fig 3-26).

2. If a new maxillomandibular relationship needs to be registered, a bite record can be made placing Kerr's impression compound or a sheet of foil sandwiched between two sheets of wax over the posterior teeth in the waxed denture (Fig 3-27). The impression material must be soft enough for the teeth to make indentations. Contact with the opposing teeth must be avoided.

3. The practitioner can readily compensate for any extra elevation of this record when the mandibular cast is remounted on the articulator; the incisal guide pin can be raised one and a half times the "Tench" thickness. To continue with the remounting, the practitioner resets the guide pin to zero to restore the VDR.

Clinical Variations

For clinical situations involving an edentulous anterior alveolar ridge, the patient should try-in artificial teeth in the available space to explore the esthetic possibilities (Fig 3-28).

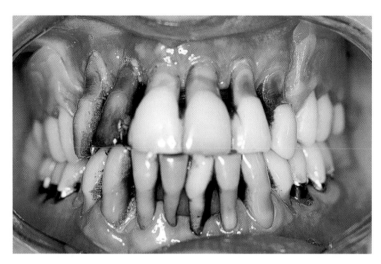

Fig 3-26 Functional try-in of the maxillary posterior waxed denture.

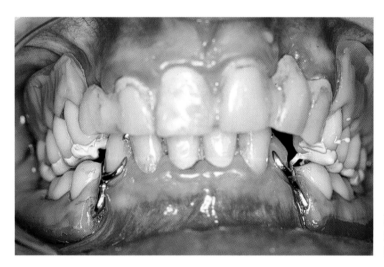

Fig 3-27 Registration of a new maxillomandibular relationship following the Tench method.

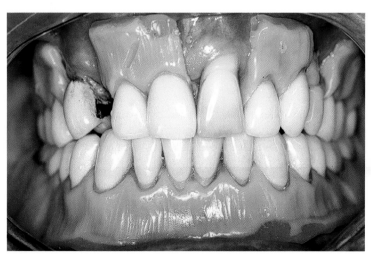

Fig 3-28 Try-in of a maxillary waxed denture with four prosthetic anterior teeth.

Finishing Details

4

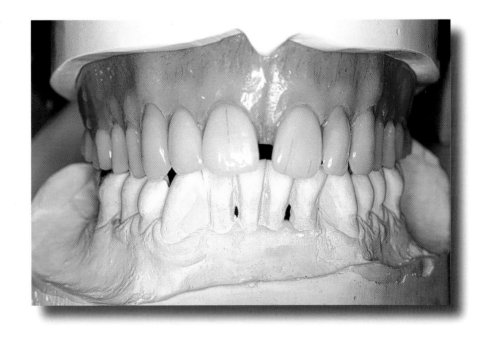

Silicone Reference Indices

Objectives
Reference indices are useful in preparing the anterior portion of the master cast in anticipation of the surgery (ie, removal of remaining anterior teeth and reduction of the alveolar ridge), which is necessary for the placement of the immediate complete denture. The two pertinent reference indices serve different purposes.

- An index of the labial region of the anterior aspect of the master cast is used to plan how much the alveolar ridge will be reduced during surgery (Fig 4-1).
- An anterior bite index helps in transferring the midincisal point and achieving the esthetic setup (Figs 4-2 and 4-3).

Materials
Silicone-based material for laboratory use.

Step-by-step laboratory procedure
1. Anterior labial index. After making two or three notches on the side wall of the master cast, the practitioner takes a silicone impression of its labial surface, including teeth, alveolar process, depth of the mucobuccal fold, and base of the cast, extending laterally to the posterior waxed denture. Following cast preparation (see the next section), the clinician can easily reposition the index, guided by unchanged areas and the notches. In this way, the index quantifies the amount of tooth and bone structure that needs to be adjusted or reduced.
2. Anterior bite index. When the articulator is closed after having silicone placed over the anterior teeth of the mandibular cast, the maxillary teeth will leave bite marks. Once the bite index is established, the practitioner trims the index symmetrically in all dimensions.

The anterior bite index is used for the transfer of the midincisal point and for execution of the esthetic setup.

> On the trimmed superior surface of the index, the practitioner marks the precise midincisal point.

The esthetic mounting can be considered at a later point.

Clinical variations
In cases where the natural anterior teeth have satisfactory esthetics, the practitioner will want to reproduce the clinical situation as accurately as possible, and the two indices play a more significant role than usual: They help the clinician to place the artificial teeth—modified in form to resemble the originals as closely as possible—into precisely the same positions as their natural precursors (see the next section).

> Just as it useful to duplicate the cast after reduction or take an impression of the inner surface of the denture to help the surgeon visualize the desired surgical result, it is a good idea to prepare another cast duplicate before reduction, with the provisional waxed denture in place to help the technician arrange the teeth in their final esthetic positions, even if it has to be reconstructed later.

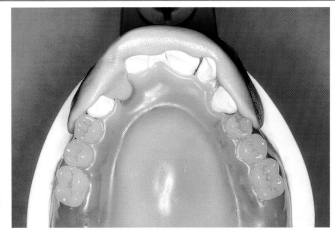

Fig 4-1 The anterior labial index, in silicone, references the original positioning of the remaining anterior teeth.

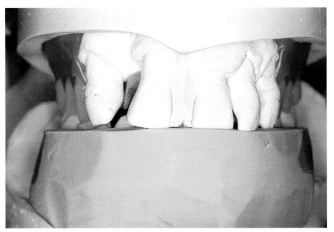

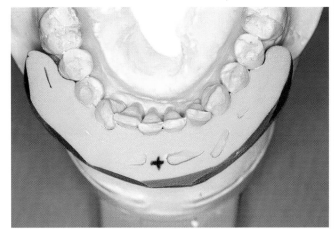

Figs 4-2 and 4-3 The anterior bite index references the sagittal and frontal location of the midincisal point.

Working Casts

Objectives

Proper preparation of a master cast, by careful anticipation of the result of wound healing, is key to successful construction of immediate complete dentures.

The master cast is refined to establish the definitive morphology for the denture-bearing surfaces, once the remaining anterior teeth have been extracted from the patient's mouth. The reshaping takes the following points into account:

- Clinical examination (eg, radiographs, periodontal probing to determine ridge height, among others (Figs 4-4 and 4-5);
- Esthetic planning, including correction of tooth malpositions and other discrepancies, and
- Prosthetic requirements including need for sufficient room between alveolar ridges, space for artifical gingiva, and others (Fig 4-6).

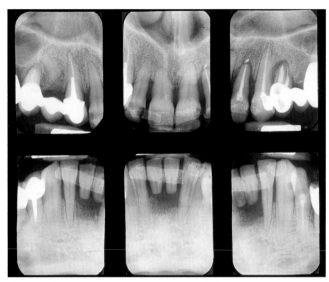

Fig 4-4 Radiographs provide a record of the alveolar and apical regions.

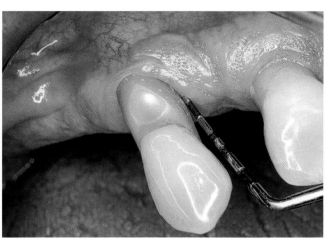

Fig 4-5 Periodontal probing can be used to estimate the height of the underlying osseous crest.

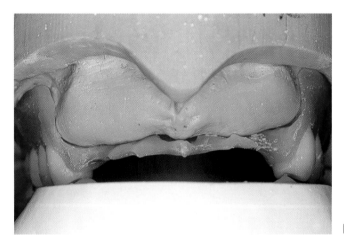

Fig 4-6 Space available for the placement of artificial gingiva.

Materials
– Knives and rotating instruments to reshape the plaster;
– Sandpaper of decreasing coarseness is used to smooth out the plaster surface.

Step-by-step clinical procedure
The practitioner first removes the teeth from the cast with a knife and then smooths out the newly formed ridge, eliminating any undercuts that would interfere with the future denture's path of insertion and removal (Figs 4-7 to 4-10).

This correction, more generous in the cervical area, diminishes progressively as the operator approaches the more apical region. No correction is made to the depth of the mucobuccal fold.

In a parasagittal section, the ridge thus prepared on the cast takes on a triangular shape. Then, the ridge details are finished by rounding off and polishing any remaining irregularities with sandpaper of decreasing coarseness (Figs 4-11 and 4-12).

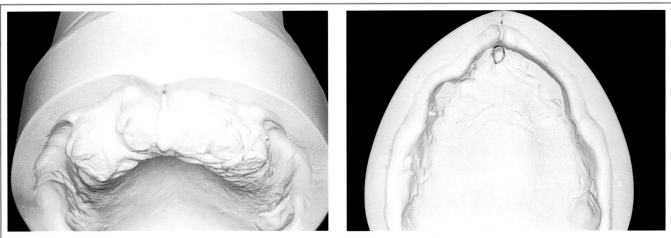

Figs 4-7 and 4-8 Preparation of the anterior portion of the cast. First the teeth are removed.

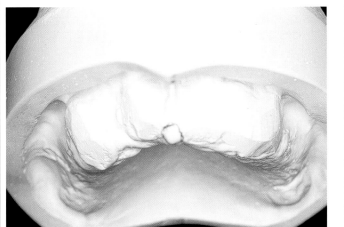
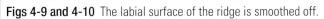
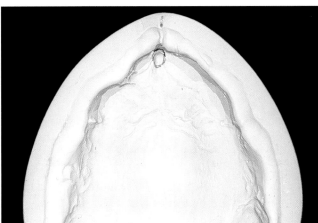

Figs 4-9 and 4-10 The labial surface of the ridge is smoothed off.

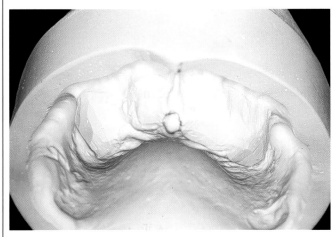
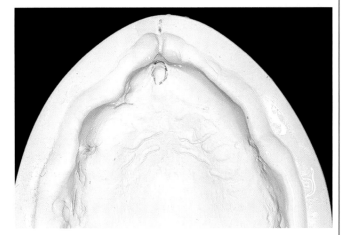

Figs 4-11 and 4-12 Irregularities are removed from the remaining anterior cast surfaces.

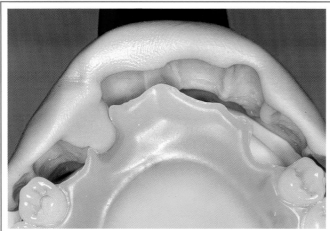
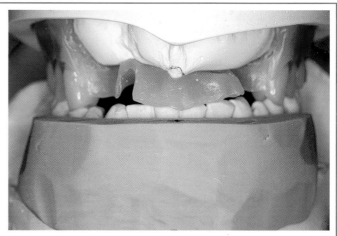

Fig 4-13 Checking the cast modification with the labial key.

Fig 4-14 Checking the cast modification with the bite key.

Practitioners should be careful not to be overly aggressive in their reduction of the anterior ridge for reception of an immediate denture because in removing too much bone, they could compromise the suitability of a possible future site for implants.

At this stage, the practitioner replaces the setup in the mouth, using the reference keys as guides, thus verifying the reduction of the anterior ridge (Figs 4-13 and 4-14). Finally, as with conventional complete dentures, the practitioner proceeds to preparing the relief for the postpalatal seal and palatal raphe.

Clinical variations

The practitioner plans the insertion and removal path of the prosthesis largely as a function of the amount of bone that is available in the supporting ridges, primarily the tuberosities. In cases where the tuberosities are not too large, it is acceptable to preserve a certain amount of retentive undercuts in anterior regions. In such cases, the denture is inserted at an angle. Still, the surgeon must find the right balance between bone retention and removal so that there will be both enough space available for minimum thickness of the denture base and support for the upper lip.

Final Mounting

Objectives

Now the dentist or technician will make the "definitive" mounting of the entire upper dental arch.

Materials

The clinician begins the esthetic mounting from the midincisal point, which had previously been marked with a cross on the bite key, by setting the artificial anterior teeth into the wax in accordance with the esthetic plan.

The functional mounting is made in conformity with the established guidelines for complete denture construction and while keeping in mind the anticipated articulation with the teeth of the opposing jaw. The clinician should have adjusted the occlusal plane of the lower jaw to a conformation that encourages the stability of the upper prosthesis, again as dictated by the established guidelines for constructing complete removable dentures. At this time, minor modifications like a simple grinding of cusps of the teeth in the opposing jaw are still possible.

Step-by-step laboratory procedure
After isolation of the corrected portion of the cast, the wax is poured to this point so that the anterior teeth can be set in (Figs 4-15 and 4-16) in strict accordance with the esthetic plan. Then, the functional setting of the posterior teeth is adjusted so that they harmonize with the anterior teeth (Fig 4-17). Even if this requires substantial adjustments, the upper posterior teeth must be positioned to articulate properly with their lower antagonists, which themselves can be adjusted at try-in time (Fig 4-18).

Final trimming and polishing of the stabilizing portion of the denture base constitute the typical final step in the construction of the maxillary setup (Figs 4-19 to 4-21).

Clinical variations
With regard to the prosthetic anterior teeth:

- If the arrangement of the anterior teeth will differ from the arrangement of the natural teeth, the prosthetic teeth are set one by one starting at the midincisal point, which had been marked on the bite key.
- If, on the other hand, the clinician plans to reproduce the arrangement of the natural teeth, the prosthetic teeth are set, one by one, in the places left by the removal of the natural teeth replicas on the cast.

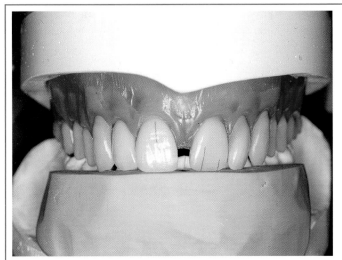

Fig 4-15 Frontal view of a completed esthetic setup of the six anterior teeth.

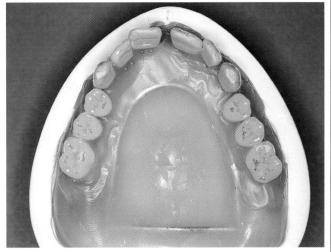

Fig 4-16 An occlusal view of a completed esthetic setup of the six anterior teeth. The posterior setup premounting of prosthetic teeth is still in place.

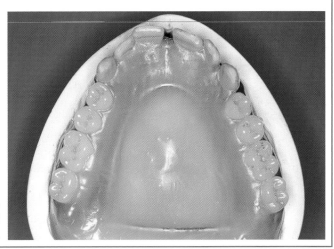

Fig 4-17 Functional setup of posterior teeth, adjusted to the anterior teeth. Note the difference as compared to the preceding figure.

After having reshaped it where needed, the clinician places each artificial tooth immediately into the place occupied by the "natural" tooth before it was removed from the cast. The reference indices and any remaining "natural" teeth are used as guides (Figs 4-22 to 4-25). The setup is completed only when all of the teeth are in place. However, to minimize the adverse reaction a new denture may elicit from friends and family, prosthetic ceramic teeth can be individually characterized to have the appearance of natural teeth.

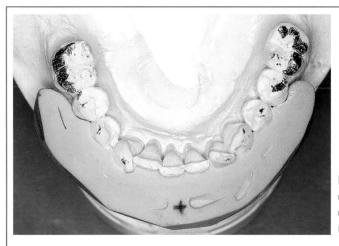

Fig 4-18 Occlusal adjustments are made to the mandibular teeth at the time of the first insertion of the denture. Equilibration must be done in line with the rules applied for mounting denture teeth.

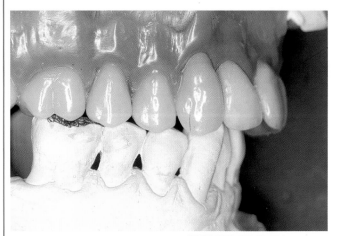
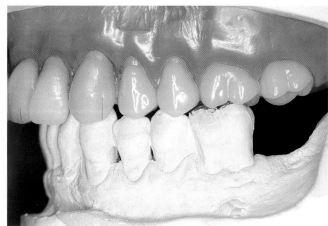
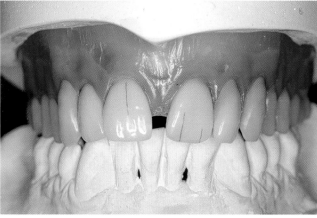

Figs 4-19, 4-20, and 4-21 Lateral and frontal views of the finalized setup of the maxillary immediate denture.

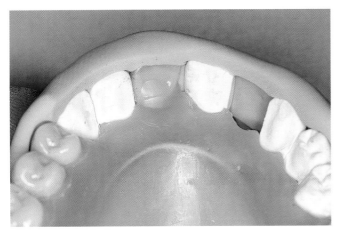

Fig 4-22 A remaining "natural" tooth on the cast has just been removed.

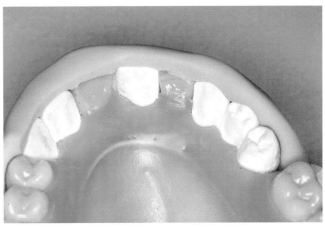

Fig 4-23 Its artifical replacement has been carefully placed precisely in the site.

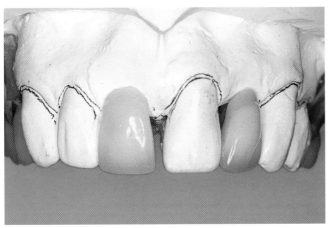

Fig 4-24 Frontal view.

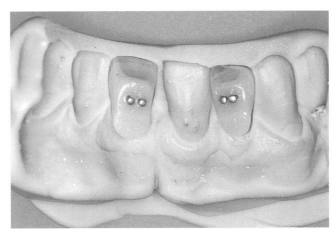

Fig 4-25 The two teeth in the labial key.

Polymerization of the Prosthesis

Objectives
This section describes the fabrication of the removable complete denture.

Materials
- The setup is flasked, and the acrylic dough forced into it is polymerized in accordance with accepted procedures for processing good quality acrylic resins that meet the highest biological and mechanical standards;
- After the acrylic is set, a final polishing and buffing will be applied to the posterior stabilizing surfaces of the denture, and a natural stippling of the anterior component will provide as life-like an appearance as possible.

Step-by-step laboratory procedure
- The wax setup is flasked (Figs 4-26 to 4-28);
- The acrylic is polymerized in accordance with the accepted guidelines for processing complete dentures.

- The teeth are equilibrated on the articulator;
- Excess is trimmed away;
- A stippled, natural appearance is imparted to the artificial gingiva;
- The application of a high polish and buffing finalizes the procedure (Figs 4-31 to 4-33).

Clinical variations

It is, of course, possible to impart a deep and realistic coloration to the artificial gingiva just as is done with any standard complete dentures.

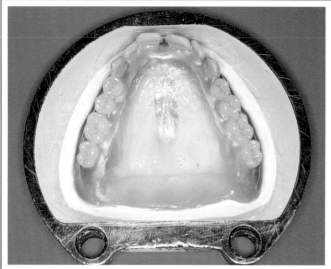

Fig 4-26 Placing the cast and wax setup in the lower flask.

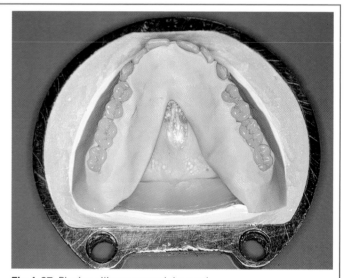

Fig 4-27 Placing silicone around the teeth.

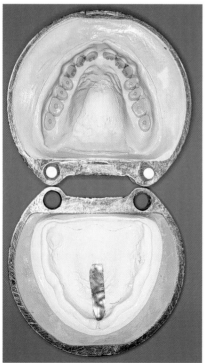

Fig 4-28 Flasking. The lower and upper component of the flask are shown after the wax was removed. The prosthetic teeth remain embedded in the upper component.

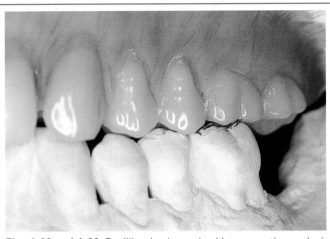
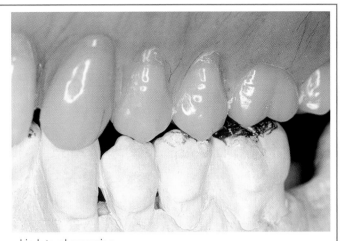

Figs 4-29 and 4-30 Equilibration in maximal intercuspation occlusion and in lateral excursion.

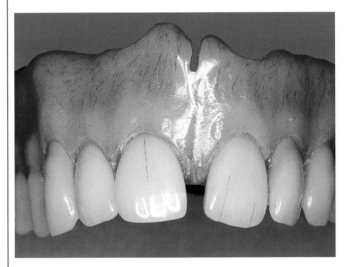
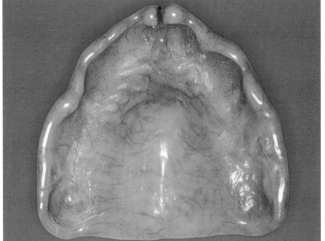

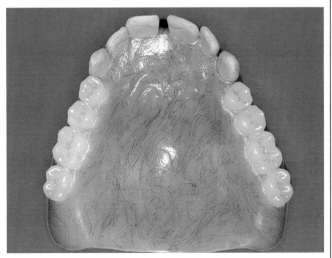

Figs 4-31, 4-32, and 4-33 A labial view of the completed prosthesis, its bearing or inner surface, and the occlusal and palatal surfaces.

Surgical Guides

Objectives
The dental laboratory aims to fabricate a surgical guide that will help the surgeon reproduce the desired clinical situation outlined previously on the working cast. The surgical guide must reproduce exactly the inner surface and the borders of the denture.

Materials
Transparent resin is used for the base. Tinted dentin-like resin is used where the teeth are reproduced for the guide.

Step-by-step laboratory procedure
• The technician blocks out the areas that would be undercuts for the denture with silicone, then boxes the guide and makes a duplicate master cast (Fig 4-34 and 4-35).
• Wax is poured into the depths of the mucobuccal fold and plate wax of even thickness is used to model the ridges and the palate;
• The surgical guide is placed in the flask (Fig 4-36);
• Polymerization of the transparent resin;
• The surgical guide is completed.

This type of surgical guide, in its most simple form, is limited to use in standard surgical procedures that require only the extraction of a few teeth and little osseous reshaping (Fig 4-37).

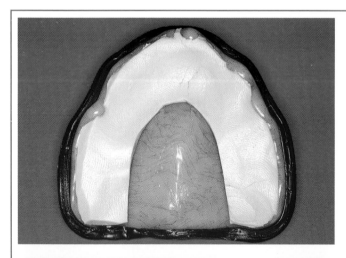

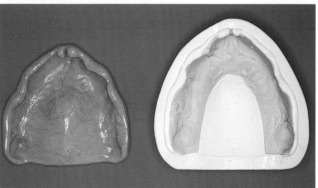

Figs 4-34 and 4-35 Fabrication of the master duplicate cast that will be used for constructing the surgical guide. The crests are molded with the hard silicone.

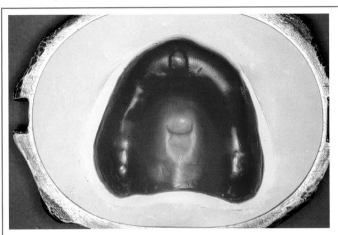

Fig 4-36 The wax-up for the simple surgical guide, made from the immediate denture, is flasked.

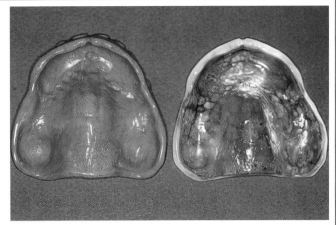

Fig 4-37 The simple surgical guide replicates the inner surface of the immediate denture.

Clinical variations

Other kinds of surgical guides can be prepared that take into account the occlusal relationships, thus ensuring that the denture base is correctly positioned at the time of surgery.

These guides are designed for complicated cases that require more extensive surgery. They are indicated in more complicated prosthetic treatments, such as trays for taking impressions to be used in functional re-adaptation and for the construction of an additional emergency replacement prosthesis.

Monobloc surgical guide with transparent teeth
This is an exact replica of the immediate prosthesis in transparent resin (Figs 4-38 to 4-40). To construct it, the technician mounts the duplicate master cast on the articulator and the prosthesis is then flasked.

This guide can be modified further to improve visibility by removal of some or all of the teeth that will be removed surgically in the mouth (Fig 4-41).

Surgical guide with removable teeth (in dentin-tinted resin)
(described by J.-M. Rignon-Bret and Roger Lerpscher)
Resin teeth are fabricated based on the denture teeth using an auto-molding technique. The teeth are arranged in blocks of three or four units. The prosthesis is placed in the lower half of the flask. Then, the blocks of resin teeth are repositioned in the appropriate space holders in the upper half of the flask (Figs 4-44 to 4-46).

The blocks of dentin-colored teeth are removable to facilitate the surgery (Fig 4-47).
But they can later be affixed to a denture base so that the unit could serve as a provisional or transitional denture (Figs 4-48 and 4-49).

This guide can also be used as an occlusal impression tray for taking impressions at a later date in case a functional re-adjustment will be necessary (see chapter 6).

In these ways, surgical guides can be used in occlusion, meaning they can assist the dentist to verify, before placing the prosthesis, that the patient's maximal intercuspal position is satisfactory (Figs 4-50 to 4-52).

And if this verification is not successful, dentists will know either:
- An error was made in establishing the intermaxillary relationship, or
- surgery will be necessary.

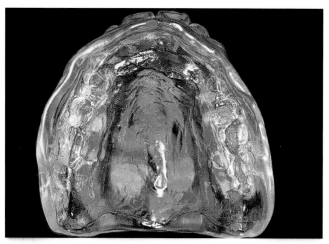

Fig 4-38 Monobloc surgical guide with transparent teeth. View of inner surface of the denture.

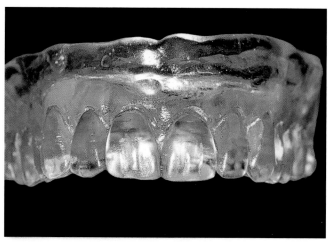

Fig 4-39 Anterior view of the monobloc surgical guide.

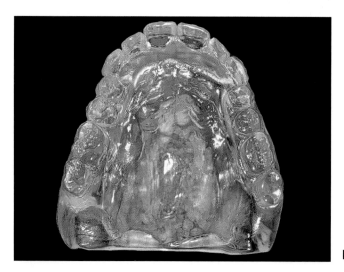

Fig 4-40 Occlusal view of the monobloc surgical guide.

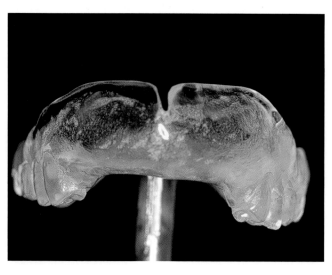

Fig 4-41 The surgical guide, with anterior teeth removed, ready to be put in occlusion.

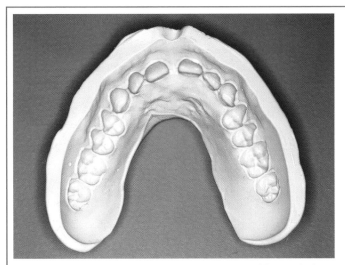

Fig 4-42 Fabrication of resin teeth by an auto-molding technique, based on a hard silicone impression of the prosthetic teeth.

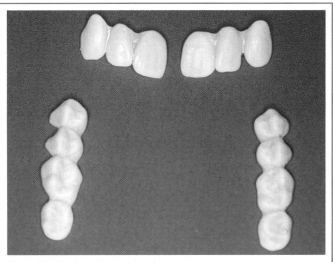

Fig 4-43 The four blocks of resin teeth.

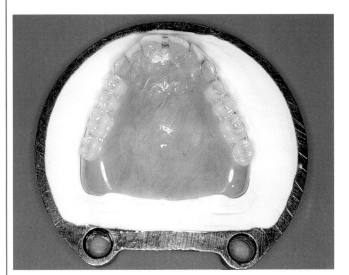

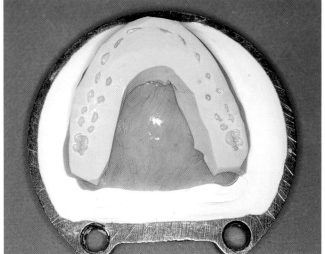

Figs 4-44 and 4-45 The prosthesis is flasked for construction of the surgical guide.

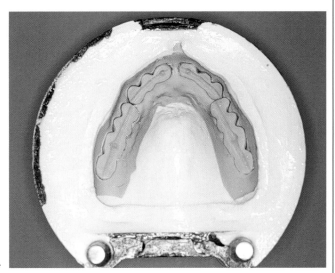

Fig 4-46 The blocks of resin teeth are repositioned.

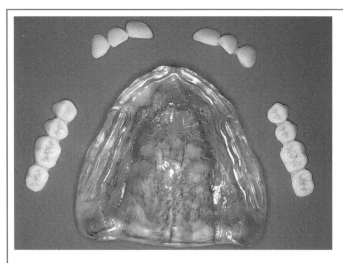
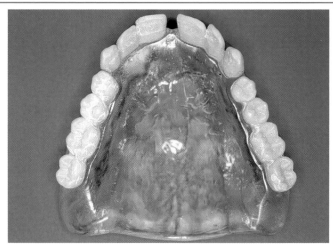

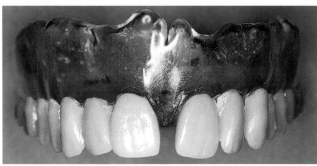

Figs 4-47, 4-48, and 4-49 Surgical guide with blocks of removable teeth.

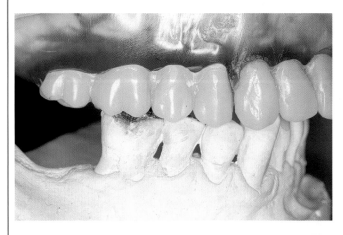
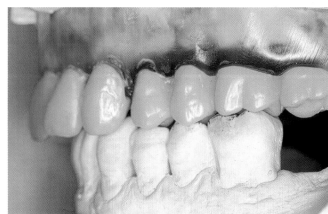

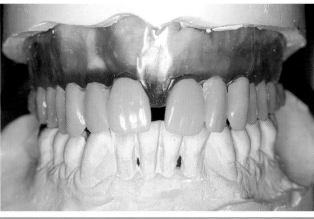

Figs 4-50, 4-51, and 4-52 Completed surgical guide in occlusion with lower cast, frontal and lateral views.

The availability of a guide for verification of the maxillomandibular relationship and potential occlusal status of the opposing mandibular teeth has also been described as useful before the surgical intervention. Such a guide deals only with posterior teeth and registers the intercuspation between the prosthetic teeth in preparation for their future natural mandibular antagonists. It is fabricated, similar to the simple surgical guide, at the time the prosthesis is flasked (Figs 4-53 to 4-56).

The ensemble of the surgical guide, the verification guide for maxillomandibular relationship and occlusal status, and the complete denture itself constitute the three components of the complete immediate denture (Figs 4-57 and 4-58).

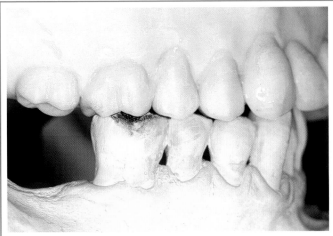
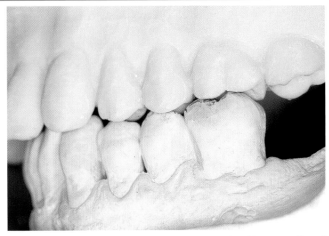

Figs 4-53 and 4-54 Guide for the verification of the maxillomandibular relationship in occlusion on the articulator. It is, in effect, a replica of the prosthesis.

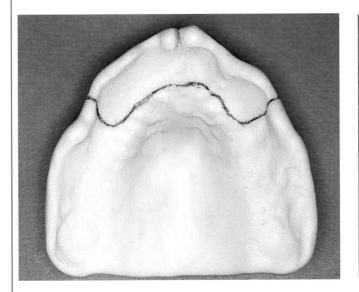
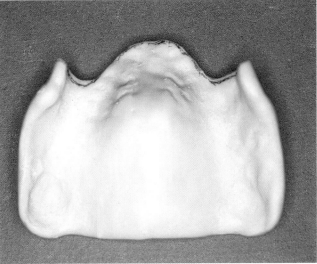

Figs 4-55 and 4-56 Cutting away of the anterior sector of the guide to assure it will fit in place before the remaining maxillary anterior teeth are extracted.

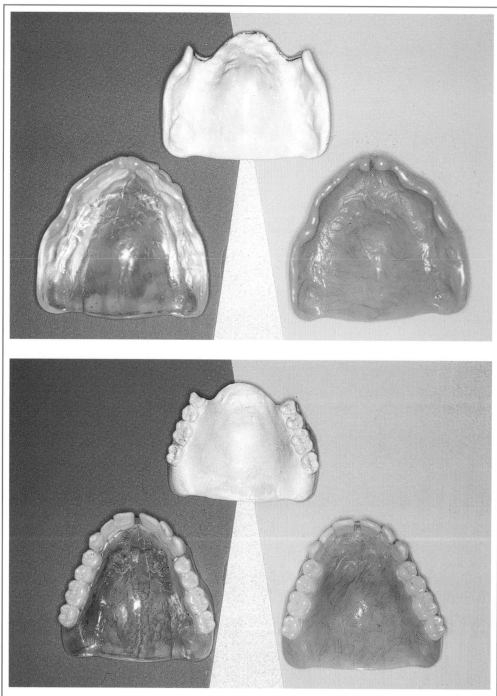

Figs 4-57 and 4-58 The prosthesis with its surgical and occlusal guides. Occlusal and inner surface views.

Delivering the Prosthesis:
Surgery and Clinical
Follow-up

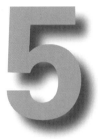

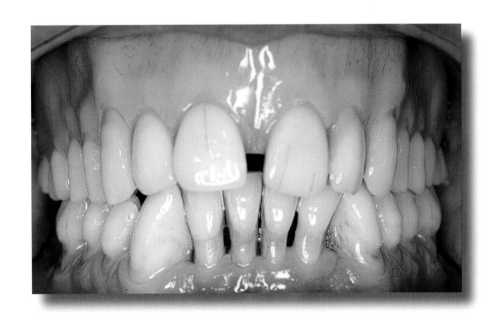

Surgery

Objectives

After removing the remaining maxillary anterior teeth, the surgeon begins to modify the underlying ridge by progressively removing bone, interspersing this remodeling with frequent checks with the surgical guide until the goal is reached.

The prosthesis can then be inserted and equilibrated.

If there is a mandibular prosthesis (or prostheses) of any kind, it should be in place at this time so that the prosthodontist can adjust the maxillary immediate denture to each of the dental units of the mandible, natural as well as prosthetic, using the prepared occlusal guide.

Materials

- Surgical guide;
- The immediate prosthesis;
- A complete or partial prosthesis for the mandible, if applicable;
- The guide for the occlusal adjustment;
- Equipment used for anesthesia, the extraction of the remaining anterior teeth, and osteo- and gingivoplasty;
- Materials for controlling and adjusting occlusion to obtain maximal intercuspation:
  - Thick articulating paper;
  - Kerr occlusal indicator wax;
  - Diamond burs and polishing cups.

Step-by-step clinical procedure

Before taking any other action, the practitioner should first verify that the mandibular prosthesis (or prostheses) is well adjusted and stable. If not, the occlusal guide should be used to balance the bite. Selective grinding is performed on the natural mandibular teeth only (Figs 5-1 to 5-4).

The actual surgical procedure begins with the injection of the local anesthetic, which should contain no vasoconstrictor. This will limit edema and allow the dentist to observe the "blanching" of the mucosa under pressure from the surgical guide.

The incision is made in the gingival sulcus and cuts through the papillae (Fig 5-5). It continues distal of the last remaining tooth on each side along the crest of the alveolar ridge. Then, a full-thickness mucoperiosteal flap is reflected, and the remaining teeth are extracted (Figs 5-6 to 5-8).

If a substantial amount of bone has to be removed in preparation of the ridge, the trimming is started by using surgical rongeur forceps on the buccal wall of the alveolar bone; if not, the next step involves the first check-up with the surgical guide.

> The areas of the mucosa that "blanch" under pressure from the guide are the ones in need of trimming. The surgeon begins this re-adjustment on the buccal wall of the alveolar ridge with surgical rongeur forceps and checks periodically with the surgical guide until the tissue blanching becomes uniform throughout, right up to the periphery of the guide, indicating that high spots have been eliminated and that the planned ridge shape has been achieved (Figs 5-9 and 5-10).

At this time, while the guide still "has its posterior teeth," the surgeon can check the occlusion in order to confirm completion of the osteoplasty (Fig 5-11).

Now the surgeon executes the mucoplasty to create a regularly shaped mucosa. The result must be confirmed with the surgical guide in place and in occlusion. Then, two or

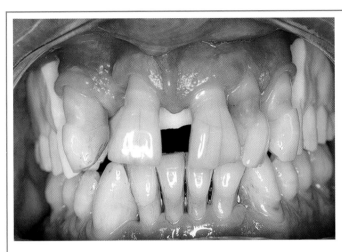

Fig 5-1 The occlusal guide is in place as the patient is readied for surgery.

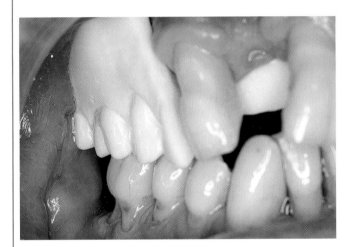

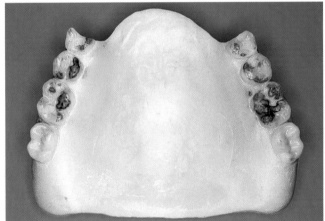

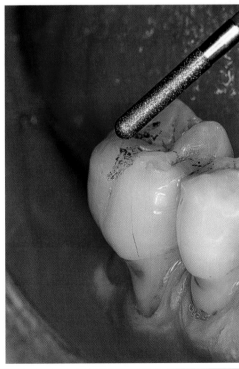

Figs 5-2, 5-3, and 5-4 The patient's natural teeth are equilibrated with the aid of the occlusal guide. Occlusal interferences are marked on the natural teeth and ground away so that the mandible will occlude properly with the maxillary denture.

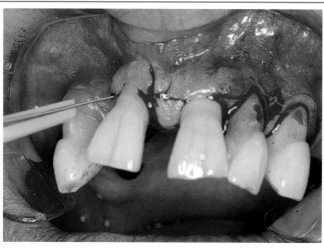
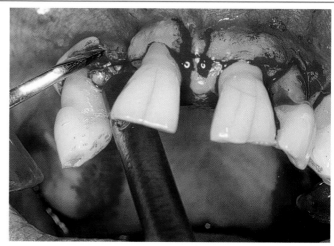

Figs 5-5 and 5-6 Incision and subsequent reflection of a vestibular flap.

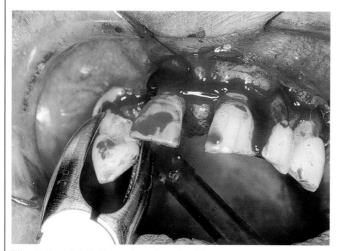
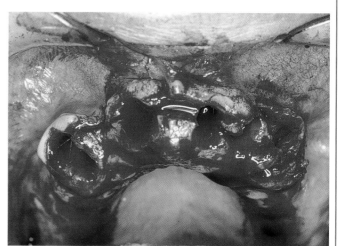

Figs 5-7 and 5-8 Extraction of teeth with appropriate forceps.

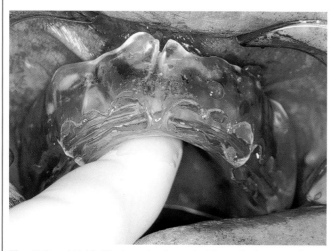
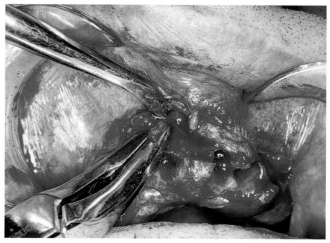

Figs 5-9 and 5-10 The bone is trimmed with surgical rongeur forceps to the extent dictated by the surgical guide. Because the tissues blanch under pressure from the guide, the surgeon is able to discern the areas that require trimming.

three sutures are placed so that the flap will not be displaced during the first one or two days after the procedure. This is done in case the patient inadvertently removes the new denture that, at this stage, is serving not just as a prosthesis but also as a surgical dressing.

The immediate complete denture is set in place (Figs 5-12 and 5-13). The patient is asked to bite on two cotton rolls to keep the denture in position and to limit the development of edema in the surgical area.

For the remainder of the appointment, the dentist shows the patient how to set the new prosthesis in place. This is followed by a few general recommendations:

• Eating a soft and nonsticky diet;
• Using analgesics as prescribed; and
• Leaving the denture in place until the follow-up visit on the next day or the day after.

It is always a good idea for the practitioner to call the patient within 24 hours of delivery of the denture.

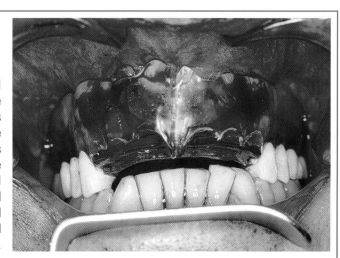

Fig 5-11 This view of an occlusal guide in occlusion indicates that the goal of the surgical intervention has been achieved. The color of the underlying mucosa reveals that it is receiving equal pressure from the guide throughout, and the occlusal relationships of the maxillary and mandibular posterior teeth are judged to conform to the pre-determined clinical standard.

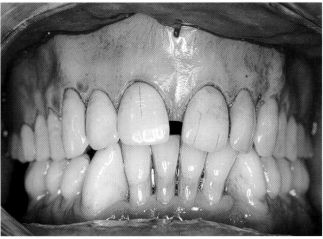

Fig 5-12 This view of the finished denture in place shows the excellent fit of the prosthetic maxillary teeth with the natural mandibular teeth.

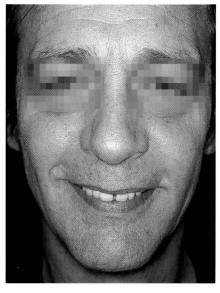

Fig 5-13 The patient smiles on the day he receives his denture.

Professor J.-C. Thibault performed the surgery for this patient.

Clinical variations

Having removable teeth associated with the surgical guide makes it useful when emergency repairs are needed or when it becomes evident at a try-in that some aspect of the maxillo-mandibular relationship requires adjustment.

The variations of the surgical guide depend on what teeth need to be extracted and what positions they occupy, the extent of their mobility, and the amount of resorption of their osseous support.

Frequently, more bone has to be removed from the region of the canine eminence than from other areas. In earlier years, surgeons would remove interdental septa with a rongeur and then fracture the external cortical plate along with its covering mucosa. This technique is no longer in use.

Immediate and Follow-up Adjustments and Equilibration

Objectives

In this step the dentist aims, if necessary, to *adjust the denture base and the occlusal relationships* to ensure the *stability of the denture* in both maximal intercuspation and all excursive movements. The denture must also be designed so that it will function satisfactorily when the patient chews or speaks.

Materials

- Fluid silicone or Kerr occlusal indicator wax;
- Thick articulating paper;
- Diamond burs, acrylic resin finishing burs, polishing cups, and other finishing materials.

And, if necessary, an appropriate instrument for removing sutures.

Step-by-step clinical procedure

Checkup visits

48 hours after denture delivery (Figs 5-14 to 5-16)

At the first visit, the practitioner personally removes the denture, which the patient had been asked to keep in place until this moment.

Next, the dentist cleans both the denture and ridge area that have been treated surgically. Using a cotton swab impregnated with hydrogen peroxide or a gauze pad dipped in chlorhexidine (Peridex) is recommended.

The sutures are removed and the denture is reinserted. Finally, the dentist checks to see if any further occlusal adjustment is needed to achieve an optimal intercuspation.

Most patients, in spite of almost universal apprehension about the experience, will not have suffered significant discomfort or other problems after receiving the prosthesis. Nevertheless, it is always advisable for the practitioner to reassure and encourage the patient at this juncture.

There are two types of lesions that may be found at this first postoperative visit. The first is an irritated labial frenum (Fig 5-17). The second is overcompression of the tissues in the region of the canine eminence, which indicates that an insufficient amount of bone had been removed at the time of surgery (Fig 5-18).

1 week to 1 month after denture delivery (Figs 5-19 to 5-24)

The practitioner adjusts the denture base to relieve any sore spots or areas of inflammation on the supporting ridges and continues occlusal equilibration to improve maximal intercuspation in centric occlusion as well as in *lateral excursive and propulsive movements*.

> The esthetic qualities of the prosthesis obviously constitute a major factor in patients' ability to accept it and to incorporate it in their lives.

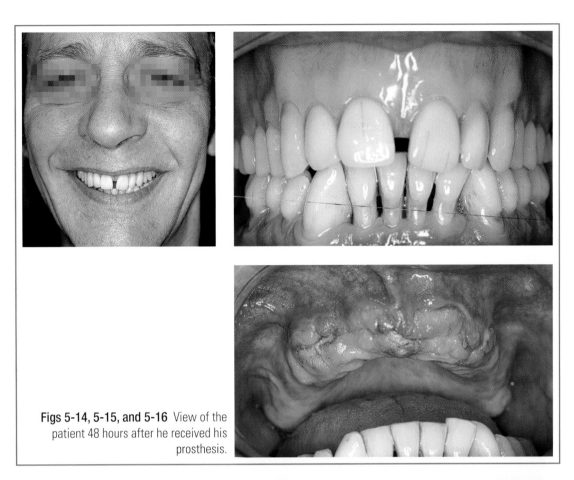

Figs 5-14, 5-15, and 5-16 View of the patient 48 hours after he received his prosthesis.

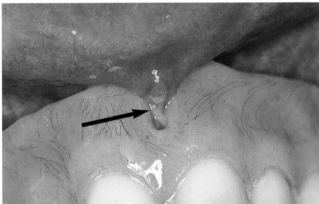

Fig 5-17 Irritation of the labial frenum.

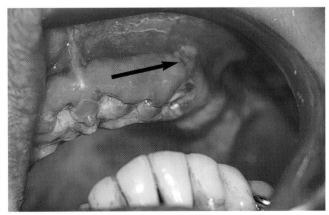

Fig 5-18 An irritated area developed in the region of the canine eminence. The surgeon had underestimated the amount of bone to remove and misjudged wound healing progress in this region.

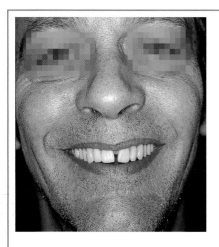
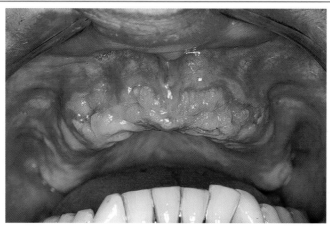

Figs 5-19 and 5-20
View of the patient 1 week after the surgical intervention.

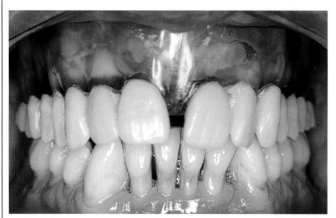
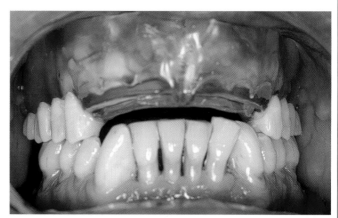

Figs 5-21 and 5-22 Check-up examination with the surgical guide in place, with and without its prosthetic anterior teeth.

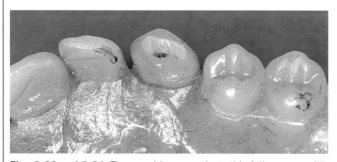
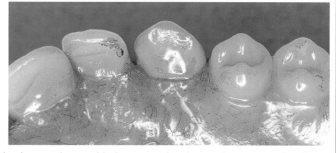

Figs 5-23 and 5-24 The practitioner conducts this follow-up equilibration in accordance with the conventional procedures appropriate for a single, complete denture construction.

The good fit and comfort provided by the new denture is of major importance to the patient, who frequently is weary of the many dental procedures that preceded the denture's delivery.

Clinical variations

All adjustments made on the immediate denture must be replicated on the removable prosthetic teeth of the surgical guide. It can be used later as an occlusally adjusted impression tray.

Reinsertion of the occlusal guide in the mouth will permit assessment of how well the tooth-bearing surfaces of the ridges have maintained their stability.

Maintenance of the Prosthesis

Objectives

A check-up visit should be scheduled for several months after delivery of the prosthesis. This check-up visit will include:

- Adjustment of the denture base to perfect its fit with the supporting ridges;
- Equilibration of the teeth for excursive movements.

If the immediate denture has been well stabilized and accepted at this time, the dentist may remind the patient of the need for another prosthesis that would be even more suitable.

Using the surgical guide in occlusion as an adapted occlusal impression tray, the practitioner can take all of the required functional re-adaptation impressions. If necessary, the procedures for articular programming and occlusion "refining" can be carried out as well.

Materials

The dentist equilibrates the teeth of the complete immediate denture using standard procedures, with medium-thickness articulating paper, and by using a semi-adjustable articulator. At this time, the surgical guide should be used to verify the absence of any unexpected osseous resorption in the surgically treated regions (Figs 5-25 to 5-28).

Step-by-step clinical procedure

From the first check-up appointment onward where the denture base is adjusted and its teeth equilibrated, it is important for the dentist to reproduce on the surgical guide any changes that were made to the working denture. An impression for restoring function can be obtained by:

- Making an occlusal index in Kerr wax or in Duralay resin so as not to lose any of the maxillomandibular relations in the course of the ongoing procedure;
- Relining the borders of the denture with a polyether material;
- Relining the denture base with a low-viscosity denture liner (Figs 5-29 to 5-31).

The patient contributes to the proper execution of this procedure by biting down to exert occlusal pressure.

Figs 5-25 and 5-26
Using the surgical guide with its removable teeth, the dentist checks to see if there has been any ridge resorption. The frontal and intraoral views show the patient, with the guide in place, several weeks after surgery.

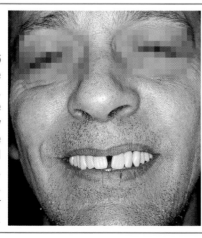
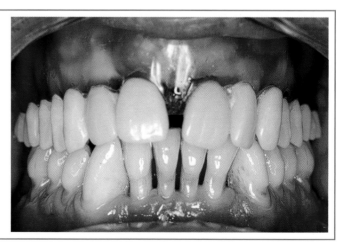

With all readings and impressions in place, a new, better-fitting, and more functional denture can be prepared for the patient. The original immediate prosthesis can be used in future emergencies.

Clinical variations

An interocclusal registration can be made with bite wax. It can be used for programming a ully adjustable articulator.

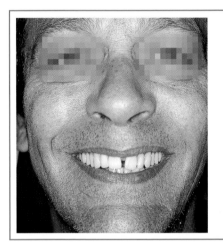
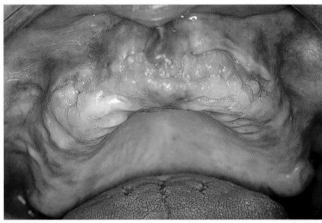

Figs 5-27 and 5-28 The immediate prosthesis has fulfilled the objectives for which it was designed: re-establishing good esthetics for the patient and preserving as much of the supporting surface of the maxillary alveolar ridges as possible.

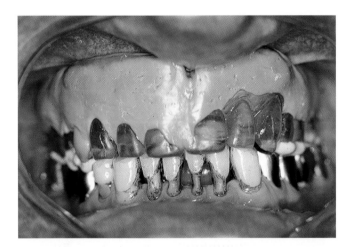
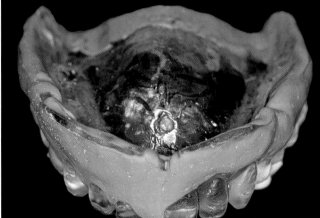
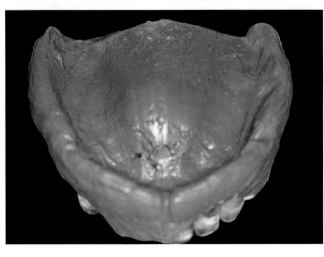

Figs 5-29, 5-30, and 5-31 The surgical guide has been used to take a functional adaptation impression. The maxillomandibular relationship has been registered in bite wax, followed by registration of the denture-bearing areas, including the inner surface of the denture and its border.

Other Clinical Situations

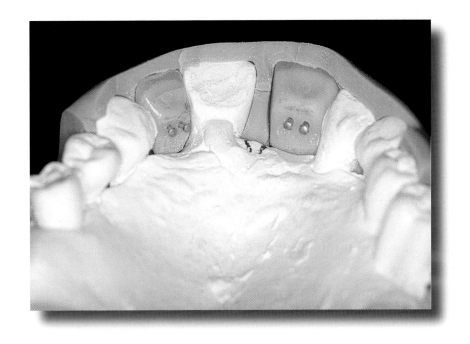

Surgery Involving Posterior Regions of the Alveolar Ridge

Situation 1

Immediate complete maxillary denture involving 14 teeth. Strictly speaking, an immediate complete denture cannot be made in this situation because the results of osseous healing are not as predictable after extraction of the posterior teeth as they are in the anterior region. While the principles of immediate complete denture construction are applied in this situation, a provisional denture, not an immediate denture, can be made. From the beginning, the patient must be informed that over time, frequent relinings, registrations of maxillomandibular relationships, and new impressions will be required to improve function (Figs 6-1 to 6-9).

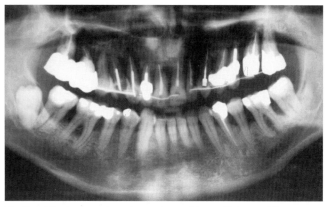

Fig 6-1 The panoramic radiograph provides sufficient evidence to support the extraction of all remaining maxillary teeth. Mandibular teeth are stabilized occlusally.

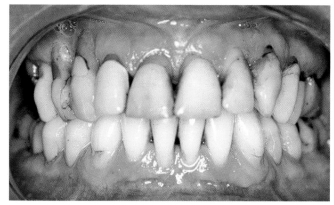

Fig 6-2 The clinical situation showing the arrangement of teeth that the young patient wanted reproduced in the planned prosthesis.

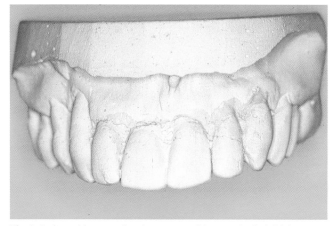

Fig 6-3 A working cast has been poured from a single initial impression. The presence of all maxillary teeth makes it impossible to take a secondary impression that includes the functional border.

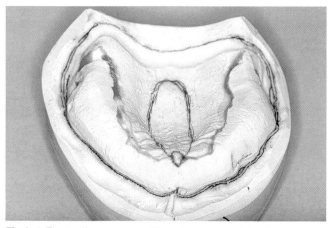

Fig 6-4 The teeth are removed from the cast, applying the principles of immediate complete denture construction. A post-dam has been carved at the junction of the hard and soft palates.

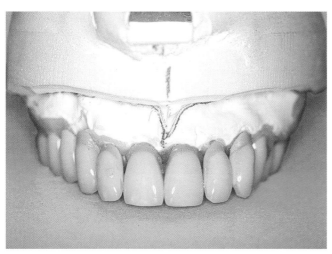

Fig 6-5 The teeth on the cast have been removed one by one and immediately replaced with an artificial tooth that mimics its predecessor as closely as possible in position, form, and shape.

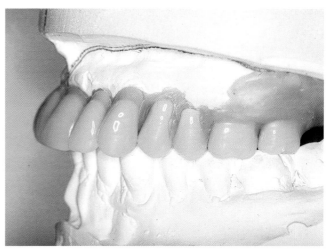

Fig 6-6 The occlusal relationship of the maxillary prosthetic teeth with the cast of the natural mandibular teeth reproduces the patient's pre-extraction intraoral situation.

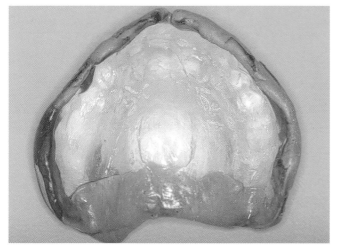

Fig 6-7 After the patient has worn the provisional denture for the 3 months required for bone healing following extractions, the surgical guide is used as a custom impression tray to take a functional impression.

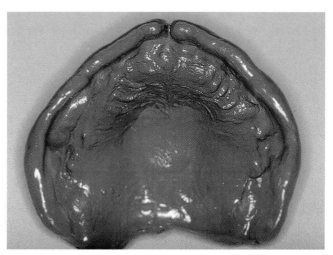

Fig 6-8 The relining impression was taken using Permlastic light, a polysulfide material.

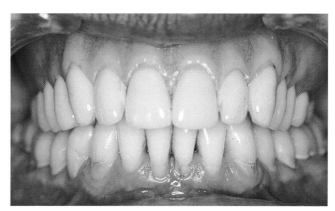

Fig 6-9 The prosthesis in place.

(Laboratory work by Roger Lerpscher.)

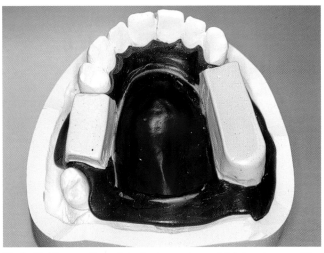

Fig 6-10 The maxillary right first premolar and third molar are still present. The denture base, with bilateral occlusal rims, assures balanced occlusal support.

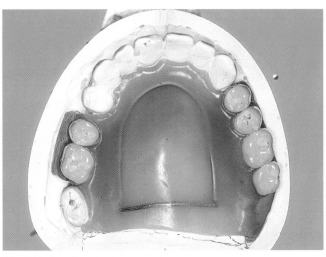

Fig 6-11 Functional setup on cast.

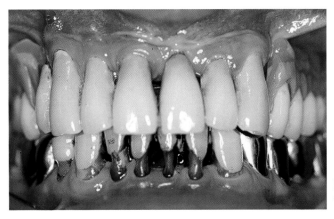

Fig 6-12 Try-in of the functional setup to register vertical dimension.

Situation 2

Remaining premolar and third molar. For this patient, the delicate task of establishing the maxillomandibular relationship is of prime importance. Its registration should be made only when occlusion between maxilla and mandible can be made at a vertical dimension that has been sufficiently increased by the occlusal blocks to eliminate any contact with its denture base or, in particular, the two natural teeth in the posterior region (Figs 6-10 to 6-12).

Situation 3

Maxillary arch reconstructed with three prostheses. A removable partial denture replaces the entire left side; a five-unit fixed partial denture has been placed on the maxillary right lateral incisor, canine, and second premolar; and the maxillary central incisors have been restored with metal ceramic crowns. The right and left prostheses are removed at each visit as steps in the construction of the complete immediate denture. Only the central incisor crowns are left in place; they serve as a guide for setting the artificial anterior teeth into the wax setup. The extraction of the maxillary right second premolar and subsequent wound healing do not affect the seating, support, or fit of the immediate denture (Figs 6-13 to 6-19).

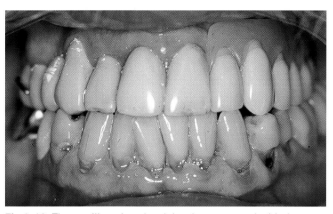

Fig 6-13 The maxillary dental arch has been restored with three types of prostheses.

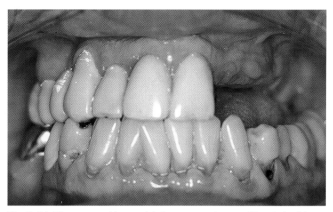

Fig 6-14 The removable partial denture on the maxillary left side has been removed.

Fig 6-15 The partial denture on the upper right side has been removed. Only the central incisors with their metal ceramic crowns are left in place to serve as guides in the esthetic setup of the denture teeth.

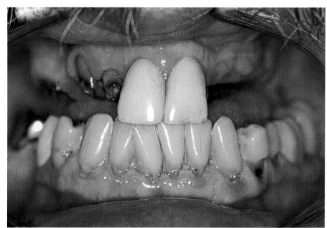

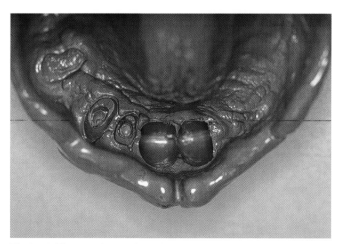

Fig 6-16 The anterior portion of the second impression shown here was taken using Permlastic light impression material.

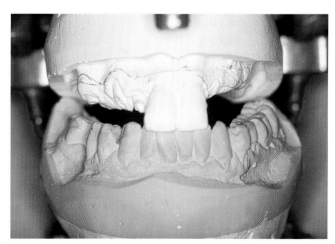

Fig 6-17 The casts mounted on the articulator. After the extraction of the second premolar has been planned on the working cast, the reshaping of the extraction can be executed using the surgical guide.

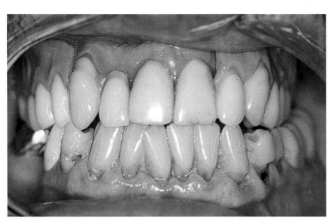

Fig 6-18 Try-in to check the function of the setup.

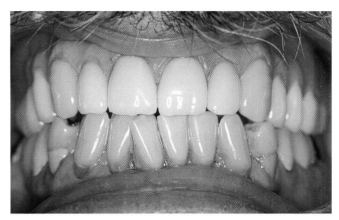

Fig 6-19 The immediate denture in place after 3 months.

Situation 4

Immediate maxillary denture replacing 10 teeth. All teeth supporting the 10-unit fixed prosthesis must be extracted in one appointment. The patient requested his new prosthesis to reproduce the appearance of the existing denture as closely as possible. During wound healing, the denture was borne bilaterally, in its center of equilibrium, by the alveolar ridges. Each artificial tooth was placed in the setup one by one into the exact position of its natural predecessor (Figs 6-20 to 6-31).

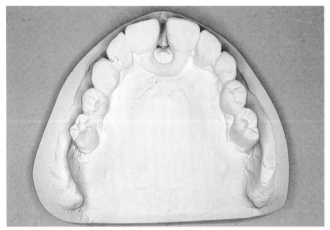

Fig 6-20 Occlusal view of the 10-unit prosthesis supported by six abutments.

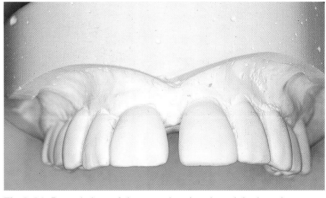

Fig 6-21 Frontal view of the cast showing the original tooth arrangement. The patient requested an identical arrangement for his denture.

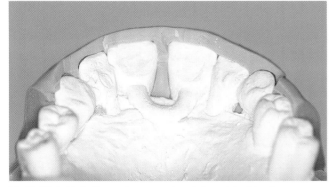

Fig 6-22 Labial silicone key reproduced the original tooth arrangement.

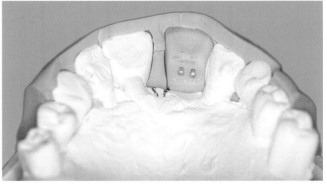

Fig 6-23 The first tooth has been removed from the cast and a prosthetic tooth set into the vacant space in the silicone key.

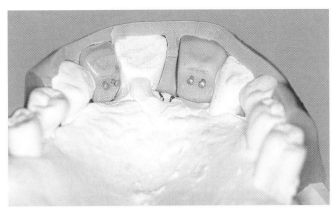

Fig 6-24 A second tooth has been placed in its silicone socket.

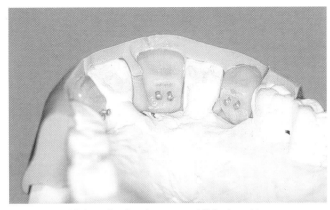

Fig 6-25 A third tooth takes its pre-established position.

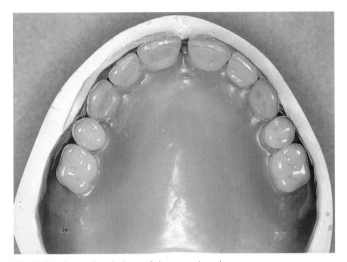

Fig 6-26 An occlusal view of the completed setup.

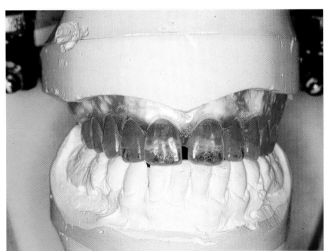

Fig 6-27 The surgical guide in occlusal position.

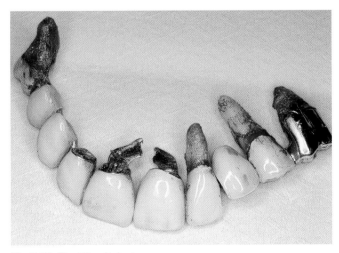

Fig 6-28 The 10-unit denture.

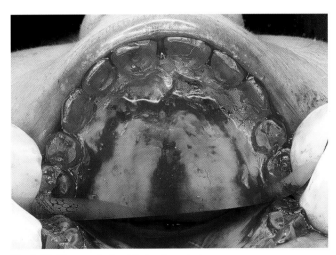

Fig 6-29 The surgical guide in place during surgery.

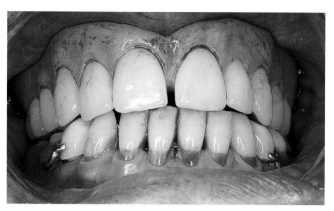

Fig 6-30 The prosthesis in place on the day of surgery.

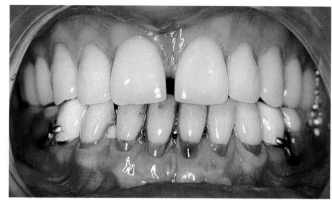

Fig 6-31 The prosthesis in place 1 month after surgery. The large amount of firm supporting ridge surface in the posterior regions assured the stability of the denture.

Situation 5

Immediate reduction of two enlarged tuberosities. Surgical guides can be designed to focus on particular regions of the supporting ridges. For this patient, a second surgical guide was fabricated with the objective of reducing the enlarged tuberosities. The reduction was limited to the hyperplastic mucosa and performed in the same appointment immediately before the teeth were extracted (Figs 6-32 to 6-35).

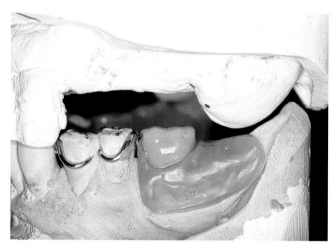

Fig 6-32 The large, bulbous tuberosity interfered with the placement of prosthetic teeth in the setup.

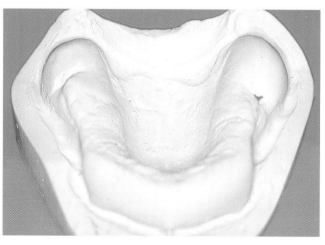

Fig 6-33 The anterior and posterior ridges of the working cast have been trimmed appropriately.

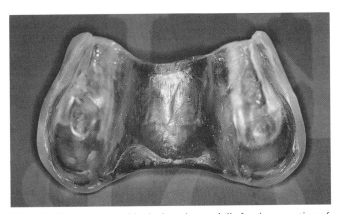

Fig 6-34 The surgical guide designed especially for the resection of the tuberosities.

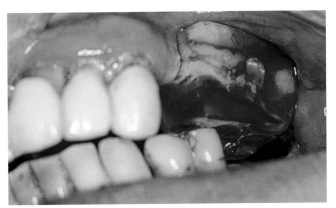

Fig 6-35 This view shows the surgical guide in place while a tuberosity is being resected, prior to tooth extraction. Then the immediate denture will be set in place with the aid of a second surgical guide.

Complete Maxillary and Mandibular Immediate Dentures

Situation 6

Of all clinical situations, this is the most delicate. The fabrication of a stable mandibular immediate denture is especially problematic because of the presence of the ever-thrusting tongue. When both jaws have to be edentulated, the resulting extreme clinical challenge must be recognized by the dentist. For this patient, dental emergencies had demanded, ultimately, extraction of all teeth. But a stable maxillomandibular relationship and excellent tissue support permitted the placement of dentures in both jaws.

After completion of wound healing, several adjustments were made to the two provisional dentures. Then, the surgical guides were used to take impressions of both jaws for a functional rehabilitation. Adjustments and equilibrations made to the two provisional prostheses at follow-up visits were exactly transferred to the individualized impression trays. Then a second set of the immediate dentures was fabricated (Figs 6-36 to 6-43).

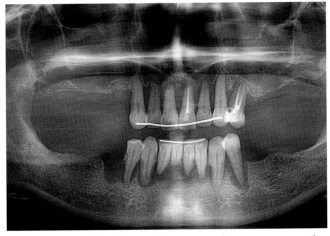

Fig 6-36 Panoramic radiograph shows extensive osseous resorption around all remaining roots in the mandible and maxilla. The vast resorption of the ridges in the posterior regions resulted in a space between denture and supporting structures that seriously compromised the stability of the prostheses.

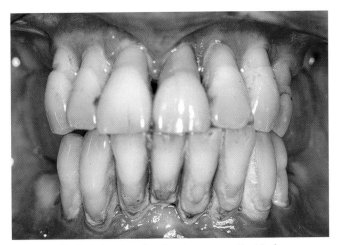

Fig 6-37 Clinical situation showing the same patient before extraction of the teeth.

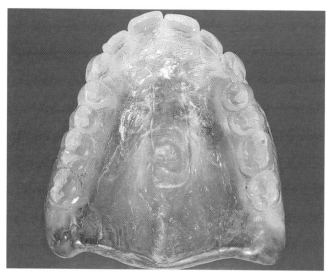

Fig 6-38 Maxillary surgical guide.

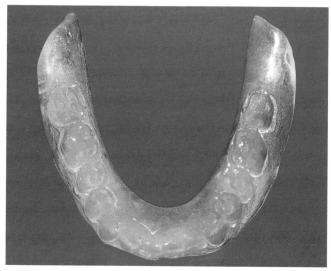

Fig 6-39 Mandibular surgical guide.

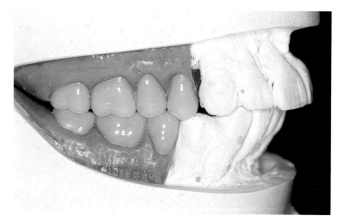
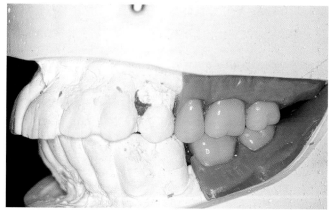

Figs 6-40 and 6-41 Lateral views of the functional setup. Occlusal stability is reduced by the small number of occlusal contacts between the maxillary and mandibular teeth, which makes control of maxillomandibular relationships precarious.

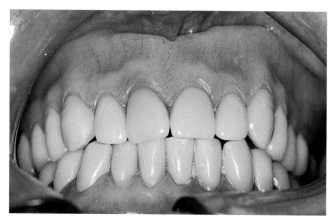

Fig 6-42 The immediate complete maxillary and mandibular prostheses in place. The principles of immediate complete denture construction were followed for taking impressions, establishing the correct relationship between the jaws, and using surgical guides. So, conditions were created that helped the patient managing the difficult transition to complete edentulousness.

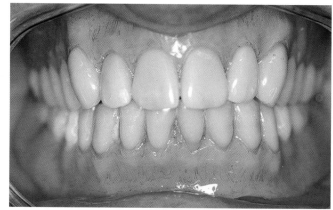

Fig 6-43 The second set of immediate prostheses in place, 3 months after delivery.

Suggested Readings

Buchard P, Apap G, Navarro M, Rignon-Bret JM. Spécial Prothèse immédiate. Cah Prothèse 1978;24:1–138.

Daas M, Pompignoli M. L'empreinte maxillaire en prothèse immédiate d'usage. Alternatives 2003;20:29–35.

Herbout B, Bertrand C, Dupuis V. Prothèse adjointe complète immédiate d'usage : Un cas clinique. Clinic 1997;9:525–529.

Herbout B, Bonifay P. Contrôle préchirurgical de l'occlusion en prothèse complète immédiate. Cah Prothèse 1999;107:29–35.

Herbout B, Postaire M. Prothèse complète immédiate d'usage. Actualisation de la technique. Cah Prothèse 2000;111:55–65.

Naser B, Postaire M, Raux D. Intérêt du porte-empreinte démontable en prothèse complète immédiate. Art et Technique Dent 1996;6:285–287.

Pompignoli M, Doukhan J-Y, Raux D. Prothèse complète: Clinique et laboratoire, vol 1, ed 2. Paris: Éditions CdP, 2000.

Pompignoli M, Doukhan J-Y, Raux D. Prothèse complète: Clinique et laboratoire, vol 2, ed 2. Paris: Éditions CdP, 2001.

Postaire M, Naser B. La prothèse immédiate d'usage. Inf Dent 1998;10:669–675.

Raux D. Guide chirurgical. Porte-empreinte en occlusion pour prothèse adjointe complète immédiate. Proth Dent 1987;7:5–12.

Rignon-Bret C, Rignon-Bret JM. Prothèse amovible complète. Prothèse immédiate. Prothèses supraradiculaire et implantaire. Paris: Éditions CdP, 2002.

Rignon-Bret JM. L'esthétique en prothèse adjointe complète, préservation ou amélioration. In: Perelmuter S. L'esthétique en odontologie. Paris: Éditions Snpmd, 1987:197–212.

Rignon-Bret JM. Les empreintes en prothèse complète immédiate (part 1). Inf Dent 1988; 16:1315–1328. (part 2);19:1689–1697.

Rignon-Bret JM. La détermination du rapport intermaxillaire en prothèse complète immédiate (part 1). Arcade antagoniste naturelle entièrement dentée. Inf Dent 1989;31:2703–2710. (part 2). Arcade antagoniste édentée. Inf Dent 1989;36:3367–3378.

Rignon-Bret JM. Le guide chirurgical duplicata à dents amovibles en prothèse complète immédiate. Cah Prothèse 1995;91:45–53.

Rignon-Bret JM. Prothèse immédiate et prothèse à barre de rétention : deux solutions prothétiques de choix pour rétablir la fonction en améliorant l'esthétique. Rev Odonto-stomatol, 1991;20:89–100.

Rignon-Bret JM, Martineau C. Prothèse complète immédiate. La rectification du modèle, l'étape chirurgicale et la pose de la prothèse. Inf Dent 1990;7:489–497.

Rignon-Bret JM, Pompignoli M. Présentation esthétique. Inf Dent 1987;32:2757–2772.

Rignon-Bret JM, Rignon-Bret C. Traitement d'un cas de dysharmonie occlusale par prothèses immédiates amovibles. Alternatives 1999;3:9–17.

Index